# Published and forthcoming Oxford Handbooks in Nursing

**Oxford Handbook of Adult Nursing**
George Castledine and Ann Close

**Oxford Handbook of Cancer Nursing**
*Edited by* Mike Tadman *and* Dave Roberts

**Oxford Handbook of Cardiac Nursing, 2e**
*Edited by* Kate Olson

**Oxford Handbook of Children's and Young People's Nursing, 2e**
*Edited by* Edward Alan Glasper, Gillian McEwing, *and* Jim Richardson

**Oxford Handbook of Clinical Skills for Children's and Young People's Nursing**
Paula Dawson, Louise Cook, Laura-Jane Holliday, and Helen Reddy

**Oxford Handbook of Clinical Skills in Adult Nursing**
Jacqueline Randle, Frank Coffey, and Martyn Bradbury

**Oxford Handbook of Critical Care Nursing**
Sheila Adam and Sue Osborne

**Oxford Handbook of Dental Nursing**
Kevin Seymour, Dayananda Samarawickrama, Elizabeth Boon, and Rebecca Parr

**Oxford Handbook of Diabetes Nursing**
Lorraine Avery and Sue Beckwith

**Oxford Handbook of Emergency Nursing**
*Edited by* Robert Crouch, Alan Charters, Mary Dawood, *and* Paula Bennett

**Oxford Handbook of Gastrointestinal Nursing**
*Edited by* Christine Norton, Julia Williams, Claire Taylor, Annmarie Nunwa, *and* Kathy Whayman

**Oxford Handbook of Learning and Intellectual Disability Nursing**
*Edited by* Bob Gates and Owen Barr

**Oxford Handbook of Mental Health Nursing, 2e**
*Edited by* Patrick Callaghan *and* Catherine Gamble

**Oxford Handbook of Midwifery, 2e**
Janet Medforth, Susan Battersby, Maggie Evans, Beverley Marsh, and Angela Walker

**Oxford Handbook of Musculoskeletal Nursing**
*Edited by* Susan Oliver

**Oxford Handbook of Neuroscience Nursing**
*Edited by* Sue Woodward and Catheryne Waterhouse

**Oxford Handbook of Nursing Older People**
Beverley Tabernacle, Marie Barnes, and Annette Jinks

**Oxford Handbook of Orthopaedic and Trauma Nursing**
Rebecca Jester, Julie Santy, and Jean Rogers

**Oxford Handbook of Perioperative Practice**
Suzanne Hughes and Andy Mardell

**Oxford Handbook of Prescribing for Nurses and Allied Health Professionals**
Sue Beckwith and Penny Franklin

**Oxford Handbook of Primary Care and Community Nursing 2e**
*Edited by* Vari Drennan *and* Claire Goodman

**Oxford Handbook of Renal Nursing**
*Edited by* Althea Mahon, Karen Jenkins, *and* Lisa Burnapp

**Oxford Handbook of Respiratory Nursing**
Terry Robinson and Jane Scullion

**Oxford Handbook of Women's Health Nursing**
*Edited by* Sunanda Gupta, Debra Holloway, *and* Ali Kubba

# Oxford Handbook of
# Mental Health Nursing

SECOND EDITION

Edited by

## Patrick Callaghan
Professor of Mental Health Nursing
University of Nottingham, UK

## Catherine Gamble
Head of Nursing, South West London and
St George's Mental Health NHS Trust;
Associate Clinical Director, Health Innovation
Network South London, UK

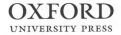

OXFORD
UNIVERSITY PRESS

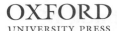

# OXFORD
## UNIVERSITY PRESS

Great Clarendon Street, Oxford, OX2 6DP,
United Kingdom

Oxford University Press is a department of the University of Oxford.
It furthers the University's objective of excellence in research, scholarship,
and education by publishing worldwide. Oxford is a registered trade mark of
Oxford University Press in the UK and in certain other countries

First Edition published 2006
Second Edition published 2015

Impression: 1

Published in the United States of America by Oxford University Press
198 Madison Avenue, New York, NY 10016, United States of America

British Library Cataloguing in Publication Data
Data available

Library of Congress Control Number: 2015941605

ISBN 978–0–19–870385–3

Printed in Great Britain by
Ashford Colour Press Ltd, Gosport, Hampshire

# Foreword

It is a great pleasure to write the foreword for this second edition of the *Oxford Handbook of Mental Health Nursing*. As the editors point out, not only has there been a major reform of how the National Health Service is organised but much has changed with regards mental health policy and practice since the publication of the first edition in 2006. The second edition captures many of these changes in the updated chapters and spells out their impact on mental health nursing. Mental health is a Government priority, not just in terms of improving and delivering excellent care but in preventing mental health problems and tackling health inequalities. There is a continual drive for mental health to have parity of esteem with physical health. At a very basic level, parity of esteem means mental health having the same value as physical health. NHS England's objective is to close the gap between people with mental health problems and the wider population, and for the first time has introduced access and waiting time standards for key mental health services as a main component of their ambition. These developments have major implications and provide opportunities for mental health nurses to play a significant part in transforming mental health care and improving the health outcomes for people with mental health problems.

Of course championing mental health is long overdue. Mental health nurses are only too well aware of the health inequalities experienced by people with mental health problems, this is exemplified by the fact that people with severe mental illness die on average 15 to 20 years earlier than other people. Mental health nurses are central to the success of the Government's ambitions and we must seize this opportunity to ensure the national commitment is translated into concrete improvements in care and treatment. This book will assist and encourage mental health nurses to achieve these ambitions, to integrate care around the service user so they receive the right care, at the right time, in the right place. By providing practical, accessible and up-to-date guidelines on the essentials of mental health nursing this book not only provides a current overview and understanding but will help shape our thinking about the design of future provision. These include, people having greater control of their own care, improved emergency access, combining health and social care, better integration of physical and mental healthcare, timely high-quality crisis care and new models of mental health liaison services.

Reading through the chapters I became aware that what is described is not just about the many changes taking place but about the advances being made in mental health nursing. Many of the advances involve working in partnership with service users and carers, taking a recovery approach, and making sure services are centred around the service user, who have more involvement in decisions and choice about their care and treatment. System changes, restructuring, reorganisation, information technology and clinical governance have all led to more efficient services, greater accountability and improvements in quality care. However, other advances are the direct results of expanding nurses' skills, knowledge and competencies, developing evidence-based interventions and measurable outcomes.

It has always seemed important to me that research activity should be directly related to informing the practice of mental health nursing, and should focus on those areas that improve health outcomes and have clear benefits for services users. I am sure nurses will find the chapters on evidence-based nursing and using research to improve practice informative and inspiring. I am sure that this section will help mental health nurses to better understand research and its role in improving health outcomes. I hope it will encourage nurses to consider taking up clinical-academic research careers. This will help expand the number of clinical academic posts and promote greater integration between clinical practice, education and research.

Although mental health is a specific field of nursing all registered nurses are expected to meet the essential mental and physical health needs of people of all ages and conditions. To provide high quality compassionate care nurses are expected to draw on a wide spectrum of attributes, knowledge and skills based on shared values and respect for human rights. The values and attitudes of professional practice are clearly articulated in the first chapter on the introduction to mental health nursing. However, anyone taking a cursory look at this handbook will be struck by the extremely complex and diverse nature of mental health nursing. The information provided required contributions from a large number of colleagues and for me raises questions around specialisation, sub-specialities and post-graduate education and training.

These issues take on even more importance for mental health nursing as therapeutic engagement and communication is the very basis of care and treatment. Each therapeutic conversation is unique and the areas of knowledge, competence and skills for mental health nurses will have different foci of expression. For example, talking to an 85-year-old woman with dementia, who also has diabetes, hypertension and arthritis (as described in Chapter 11), would require an emphasis on different competencies to someone with incapacitating social phobia who is unable to form social relationships, has difficulties in interactions with others and problems in work caused by avoidance (as described in Chapter 7).

As we go to press we await the publication of two key documents: the recommendations of NHS England's Mental Health Taskforce and the new nursing strategy. Both of these documents will have implications for mental health nursing and although we should not second guess the content, one thing we can be certain about is that whatever the recommendations, mental health nursing will be central to driving forward any changes and developments aimed at improving the quality of care and the health outcomes of people with mental health problems.

I would like to congratulate the authors and editors for producing such a welcome, comprehensive, relevant, and scholarly edition to the mental health nursing literature.

Dr Ben Thomas
Mental Health, Learning Disability and
Dementia Care Professional Officer
Strategy and External Relations Directorate
Department of Health, UK

# Preface

The second edition of the *Oxford Handbook of Mental Health Nursing* follows from the success of the first edition, published in 2006. The purpose of the book remains to provide practical, accessible, concise, and up-to-date evidence-based guidelines on the essentials of mental health nursing in one handy portable format that will appeal to busy clinicians.

Much has happened since the publication of the first edition. There have been two changes of government, two strategic plans for mental health in England, a substantial reorganization of the NHS, a revised Mental Health Act in England, four reviews of nursing, two of which concerned mental health nursing, and the implementation of a national Improving Access to Psychological Therapies (IAPT) programme. The *Diagnostic and Statistical Manual of Mental Disorders*, Fifth Edition (DSM-5) has been published, inviting acclaim and approbation. Various inquiries into care in the NHS have highlighted the need for nurses to remain compassionate, caring, and competent, to have the courage to stand up for, and be committed to, the highest standards of care, and to demonstrate effective communication skills. Amid these changes the prevalence of mental disorders has increased across the world to the extent that it is estimated that around 1 in 4 people experience mental health problems. Mental illness is predicted to be the second commonest cause of disability worldwide by the end of this decade. The publication of the second edition of the *Oxford Handbook of Mental Health Nursing* to reflect these changes is therefore timely.

Each chapter of this second edition has been reviewed and where necessary updated to reflect the changes in our knowledge and understanding of mental health nursing.

Notwithstanding the changes that we have made to the second edition, we have retained the format that allows readers quick and easy access to the information in a user-friendly manner. A notable amendment to the second edition is the change of one of the editors. Helen Waldock has now retired from mental health nursing after a significant and distinguished career. We wish to express our huge thanks to Helen for her work on the first edition, and we wish her a long, happy, and healthy retirement.

It is our intention that the second edition of the book will be read by mental health nurses, students, and others working across and within mental health services who are committed to improving the care of people using these services, and their carers and families. We hope that the book will enable mental health nurses to continue to uphold the finest traditions of the profession in working collaboratively and in partnership with people to help them to lead a meaningful and satisfying life free from incapacitating mental distress.

PC and CG

# Contents

# Contributors to the second edition

**Marie Armstrong**
Nurse Consultant, Nottingham Child and Adolescent Mental Health Services (CAMHS), UK

**Julie Attenborough**
Lecturer in Mental Health Nursing (Substance Abuse), City University, London, UK

**Len Bowers**
Professor of Psychiatric Nursing, King's College, London, UK

**Geoff Brennan**
Executive Director, Star Wards, London, UK

**Dan Bressington**
Assistant Professor, School of Nursing, The Hong Kong Polytechnic University, Hong Kong

**Sarah Eales**
Lecturer in Mental Health, Senior Lecturer in Mental Health Nursing, Bournemouth University, UK

**Richard Gray**
Assistant Executive Director (Nursing) Research, HMC Qatar; Professor of Nursing, University of Calgary; Visiting Professor, The Hong Kong Polytechnic University, Hong Kong

**Ben Hannigan**
Co-Director of Postgraduate Research, Mental Health and Learning Disabilities Team, Cardiff University, UK

**Carl Holvey**
Principal Clinical and Deputy Chief Pharmacist, Pharmacy Department, South West London and St George's Mental Health NHS Trust, UK

**Julia Jones**
Reader, School of Health Sciences, City University, London, UK

**Sarah Kendal**
Principal Lecturer and Head of Division of Mental Health and Learning Disability, Huddersfield University, UK

**Karina Lovell**
Director of Research and Professor of Mental Health, School of Nursing, Midwifery and Social Work, University of Manchester, UK

**Joanne Lymn**
Director of Research, School of Health Sciences, University of Nottingham, UK

**Patricia McBride**
Director of Undergraduate Programmes, School of Health Sciences, University of Stirling, UK

**Edward McCann**
Assistant Professor, School of Nursing and Midwifery, Trinity College Dublin, Ireland

**Maria Michail**
Senior Research Fellow in Mental Health, School of Health Sciences, University of Nottingham, UK

**Jean Morrissey**
Lecturer, School of Nursing and Midwifery, Trinity College Dublin, Ireland

**Madeline O'Carroll**
Acting Programme Manager (Mental Health), School of Health Sciences, Nursing, City University, London, UK

**Sara Owen**
Faculty of Health, Life and Social Sciences, University of Lincoln, UK

**Julie Repper**
Director of Improving Recovery through Organisational Change (ImROC), UK

**Dave Richards**
Professor of Mental Health Services Research and NIHR Senior Investigator, Exeter University, UK

**Paul Rogers**
Chair of Forensic Nursing, Faculty of Health, Sport and Science, University of Glamorgan, UK

**Peter Ryan**
Professor of Mental Health, School of Health and Education, Middlesex University, London, UK

**Alan Simpson**
Professor of Collaborative Mental Health Nursing, School of Health Sciences, City University, London, UK

**Allison Tennant**
Peaks Unit, Rampton Hospital, Retford, UK

**Malcolm Wandrag**
Lecturer, School of Health Sciences, City University, London, UK

**Richard Whittington**
Professor of Mental Health, Institute of Psychology, Health and Society, University of Liverpool, UK

With thanks to the editor of the first edition:

**Helen Waldock**
Health and Social Care Advisory Service, London, UK

Specialist reviewer:

**Ian Hulatt**
Professional Lead for Mental Health, Nursing Department, Royal College of Nursing, London, UK

# Contributors to the first edition

Jane Alexander

Neil Brimblecombe

Jenny Cobb

Tina Coldham

Scott Durairaj

Chris Flood

Cathe Gaskell

Neil Gordon

Paul Hammersley

Androulla Johnstone

Mariya Limerick

Shameen Mir

Soo Moore

Jan Murray

Peter Phillips

Rosemary Russell

Iain Ryrie

Phillippa Sully

Lynny Turner

Helen Waldock

# Symbols and abbreviations

| | |
|---|---|
| ↓ | decreased |
| ↑ | increased |
| ➔ | cross reference |
| ℳ | mouse symbol |
| AADD | adult attention deficit disorder |
| ADHD | attention deficit hyperactivity disorder |
| ADOS | Autism Diagnostic Observation Schedule |
| AIMS | Abnormal Involuntary Movement Scale |
| AMHP | Approved Mental Health Professional |
| AOT | assertive outreach team |
| APA | American Psychiatric Association |
| ASW | approved social worker |
| BA | behavioural activation |
| BAI | Beck Anxiety Inventory |
| BAS | Barnes Akathisia Scale |
| BAVQ | Beliefs About Voices Questionnaire |
| BDI | Beck Depression Inventory |
| BME | black and minority ethnic |
| BMI | body mass index |
| BNF | *British National Formulary* |
| bpm | beats per minute |
| BPRS | Brief Psychiatric Rating Scale |
| BSQ | Body Shape Questionnaire |
| BVC | Brøset Violence Checklist |
| CAMHS | Child and Adolescent Mental Health Services |
| CAMI | Carers' Assessment of Managing Index |
| CASP | Critical Appraisal Skills Programme |
| CBT | cognitive behavioural therapy |
| CCG | clinical commissioning group |
| CCNAP | Community Care Needs Assessment Project |
| CFS | chronic fatigue syndrome |
| CMHT | community mental health team |
| CMP | clinical management plan |
| CNO | Chief Nursing Officer |
| COP | Code of Practice |
| CORP | Clinical Outcome Review Programme |

| CPA | Care Programme Approach |
| --- | --- |
| CQC | Care Quality Commission |
| CQUIN | Commissioning for Quality and Innovation |
| CREST | Clinical Resource Efficiency Support Team |
| CTO | Community Treatment Order |
| DBRS | Dangerous Behaviour Rating Scale |
| DBS | Disclosure and Barring Service |
| DBT | dialectic behavioural therapy |
| DOLS | deprivation of liberty safeguards |
| DPA | Data Protection Act |
| DSH | deliberate self-harm |
| DSM-5 | *Diagnostic and Statistical Manual of Mental Disorders,* *Fifth Edition* |
| DSPD | dangerous and severe personality disorder |
| EAT | Eating Attitudes Test |
| ECT | electroconvulsive therapy |
| EDI-3 | Eating Disorders Inventory—3 |
| EE | expressed emotion |
| ENDS | Evaluation of Nursing Documentation Schedule |
| EPDS | Edinburgh Postnatal Depression Scale |
| EPSE | extrapyramidal side effects |
| FDA | US Food and Drug Administration |
| FRASE | Falls Risk Assessment Scale for the Elderly |
| GABA | gamma-aminobutyric acid |
| GAD | generalized anxiety disorder |
| GASS | Glasgow Antipsychotic Side-effect Scale |
| GHQ | General Health Questionnaire |
| GMC | General Medical Council |
| GSH | guided self-help |
| HADS | Hospital Anxiety and Depression Scale |
| HCR-20 | Historical, Clinical, Risk Management 20-item scale |
| HoNOS | Health of the Nation Outcome Scale |
| HQIP | Healthcare Quality Improvement Partnership |
| HT | humanistic therapy |
| ICD | International Classification of Disease |
| IPT | interpersonal psychotherapy |
| ISA | Independent Safeguarding Authority |
| IT | information technology |
| JCP | joint crisis plan |
| LMHS | liaison mental health services |

| LUNSERS | Liverpool University Neuroleptic Side Effect Rating Scale |
| MCA | Mental Capacity Act |
| MHA | Mental Health Act |
| MHO | Mental Health Officer |
| MHRA | Medicines and Healthcare products Regulatory Agency |
| MHRT | Mental Health Review Tribunal |
| MHT | Mental Health Tribunal |
| MI | motivational interviewing |
| MMSE | Mini Mental State Examination |
| MRSA | methicillin-resistant *Staphylococcus aureus* |
| MWC | Mental Welfare Commission |
| NARI | noradrenaline reuptake inhibitor |
| NaSSA | noradrenergic and specific serotonergic antidepressant |
| NCAPOP | National Clinical Audit and Patient Outcomes Programme |
| NERS | Nurses' Evaluation Rating Scale |
| NHS | National Health Service |
| NICE | National Institute for Health and Care Excellence |
| NMC | Nursing and Midwifery Council |
| NOSIE | Nurses' Observation Scale for Inpatient Evaluation |
| NSF | National Service Framework |
| OCD | obsessive–compulsive disorder |
| PANSS | Positive and Negative Syndrome Scale |
| PCL-R | Psychopathy Checklist–Revised |
| PD | personality disorder |
| PHC | Physical Health Check |
| PM | postmodern |
| PSI | psychosocial interventions |
| PSYRATS | Psychotic Symptom Rating Scales |
| PTSD | post-traumatic stress disorder |
| QRP | Quality and Risk Profile |
| RAID | Rapid Assessment Interface and Discharge |
| RCT | randomized controlled trial |
| REM | rapid eye movement |
| RMO | responsible medical officer |
| ROT | reality orientation therapy |
| SAM | Suicide Assessment and Management |
| SAS | Simpson Angus Scale |
| SCANS | Setting Conditions for Anorexia Nervosa Scale |
| SCIE | Social Care Institute for Excellence |
| SCOFF | Sick, Control, One, Fat, Food |

| SCT | Supervised Community Treatment |
| SEC | Side Effects Checklist |
| SES | Self-Esteem Scale |
| SF-12 | Short Form-12 |
| SFS | Social Functioning Scale |
| SMI | serious mental illness |
| SNRI | serotonin and noradrenaline reuptake inhibitor |
| SOAS | Staff Observation Aggression Scale |
| SP | supportive psychotherapy |
| SSRI | selective serotonin reuptake inhibitor |
| STRATIFY | St Thomas's Risk Assessment Tool in Falling Elderly Inpatients |
| TCA | tricyclic antidepressant |
| TOC | Triangle of Care |
| UK | United Kingdom |
| VRAG | Violence Risk Appraisal Guide |
| WHO | World Health Organization |
| WRAP | Wellness Recovery Action Plan |

# Introduction to mental health nursing

# Mental health and well-being in the global context

Mental illness is now one of the most common disorders affecting people worldwide. Neuropsychiatric diseases account for 13% of the global burden of disease, yet only 6% of financial resources are allocated to mental health.[1] The consequences of these disorders are estimated to cost approximately US$ 16.1 trillion in loss of productivity, have severe impacts on quality of life, arrest social development, and increase the risk of suicide, stigma, discrimination, inequity, and medical problems such as diabetes and cardiovascular disorders.[2,3]

The key messages from the World Health Organization (WHO) *Mental Health Atlas*[1] are as follows:

- There are insufficient resources to treat mental illness. Spending on mental health is less than US$ 2 per person per year in high-income countries, and less than 25 cents in low-income countries.
- For around 50% of the world's population there is one psychiatrist per 200,000 people.
- In 92% of high-income countries there is mental health legislation covering the care of people with mental disorders; the corresponding figure for low-income countries is 36%.
- Community mental health facilities are 58 times more likely to exist in high-income countries.
- Service user/consumer organizations exist in 83% of high-income countries, compared with 49% of low-income countries.
- Around 67% of mental health spending is directed towards inpatient services.
- There has been a modest decrease in the number of inpatient beds globally.
- Around 60% of countries have a national mental health policy, and around 71% have a mental health plan.
- For every 100,000 members of the world's population there are 0.61 outpatient services, 0.05 day treatment services, 0.01 community residential services, and 0.04 psychiatric hospitals.
- Follow-up mental health care is provided by 32% of countries; the higher an individual's socio-economic status, the more likely they are to receive follow-up care.
- Psychosocial interventions are provided in 44% of countries, and again this is linked to socio-economic status, with those in the lower-income groups being less likely to receive psychosocial interventions.
- Nurses represent the largest proportion of professionals providing mental health care; the median average number of nurses working in mental health per 100,000 members of the population is 5.8, more than all the other professional groups combined.
- The mean expenditure on medications for mental health and behavioural disorders is around US$ 6.81 per person, although it is estimated that in reality this figure is lower, as only 27% of countries reported data on this issue to *The Mental Health Atlas*.

The WHO *Mental Health Action Plan for 2013–2020*[4] aims to promote mental well-being, prevent mental disorders, and reduce mortality and morbidity in individuals with mental health problems. The action plan proposes six cross-cutting principles (see Table 1.1).

**Table 1.1** Cross-cutting principles proposed by the WHO *Mental Health Action Plan for 2013–2020*[4]

| Principle | Target |
| --- | --- |
| Universal health coverage | Regardless of age, gender, socio-economic status, race, ethnicity, or sexual orientation, and following the principle of equity, persons with mental disorders should be able to access, without the risk of impoverishing themselves, essential health and social services that enable them to achieve recovery and the highest attainable standard of health |
| Human rights | Mental health strategies, actions, and interventions for treatment, prevention, and promotion must be compliant with the Convention on the Rights of Persons with Disabilities and other international and regional human rights instruments |
| Evidence-based practice | Mental health strategies and interventions for treatment, prevention, and promotion need to be based on scientific evidence and/or best practice, taking cultural considerations into account |
| Life course approach | Policies, plans, and services for mental health need to take account of health and social needs at all stages of the life course, including infancy, childhood, adolescence, adulthood, and older age |
| Multisectoral approach | A comprehensive and coordinated response for mental health requires partnership with multiple public sectors, such as health, education, employment, judicial, housing, social, and other relevant sectors, as well as the private sector, as appropriate to the country situation |
| Empowerment of persons | Persons with mental disorders and psychosocial disabilities should be empowered and involved in mental health advocacy, policy, planning, legislation, service provision, monitoring, research, and evaluation |

## References

1 World Health Organization. *The Mental Health Atlas*. World Health Organization: Geneva, 2011.
2 Ganju V. Non-communicable diseases and the mental health gap: what is to be done. *International Journal of Psychiatry* 2012; 9: 79–80.
3 Bass JK et al. A United Nations General Assembly special session for mental, neurological and substance use disorder: the time has come. *PLOS Medicine* 2012; 9: e1001159.
4 World Health Organization. *Mental Health Action Plan for 2013–2020*. World Health Organization: Geneva, 2013. ℘ http://apps.who.int/iris/bitstream/10665/89966/1/9789241506021_eng.pdf

# Strategic visions for mental health nursing

## Introduction

Since the publication of the first edition of this Handbook in 2005, four reports have been produced that have outlined a vision for nursing, two of which focused on mental health nursing.

## The Chief Nursing Officer's (CNO) review of mental health nursing in England (2006)

This CNO review[5] made recommendations for practice and education, with promoting people's recovery at its core. As part of the review the Department of Health published good practice guidance for pre-registration mental health nurse education,[6] and a 'self-assessment toolkit' to enable trusts to assess progress in implementing the review recommendations.[7] The review emphasized three main themes and a number of sub-themes:

*Putting values into practice*
- *Values*—promote a culture that values and respects the diversity of individuals, and enables their recovery.

*Improving outcomes for service users*
- *Communication*—use a range of communication skills to establish, maintain, and manage relationships with individuals who have mental health problems, their carers, and key people involved in their care.
- *Physical care*—promote physical health and well-being for people with mental health problems.
- *Psychosocial care*—promote mental health and well-being, enabling people to recover from debilitating mental health experiences and/or achieve their full potential, supporting them to develop and maintain social networks and relationships.
- *Risk and risk management*—work with individuals with mental health needs in order to maintain their health, safety, and well-being.

*A positive, modern profession*
- *Multidisciplinary and multi-agency working*—work collaboratively with other disciplines and agencies to support individuals to develop and maintain social networks and relationships.
- *Personal and professional development*—demonstrate a commitment to the need for continuing professional development and personal supervision activities, in order to enhance knowledge, skills, values, and attitudes needed for safe and effective nursing practice.

## The Chief Nursing Officer's (CNO) review of mental health nursing in Scotland (2006)

A similar review was conducted in Scotland,[8] and it emphasized three areas:

*Culture and values: strengthening the climate of care*
- Mental health nursing is about caring for people and their significant others, spending time with them, and developing sound interpersonal relationships.
- Mental health nursing is rights based, with a person-centred focus that promotes values- and principles-based practice.
- Recovery principles should be adopted.
- Models of care should be adopted that are relationship based and use contact time to foster recovery.

*Practice and services*
- Prioritize the focus of care towards acute inpatient, crisis care, and home treatment services.
- Adopt the strengths-based approach to recovery.
- Prepare mental health nurses to work effectively with older adults.
- Enhance the role of mental health nurses in early intervention and risk assessment.
- Develop the role of mental health nurses in health promotion, health improvement, and reducing inequalities.

*Education and development*
- Develop a national framework to attract the right people into the profession.
- Emphasize continuing professional development.
- Involve service users and carers in all aspects of mental health nursing.
- Promote the development of mental health support workers.
- Develop and embed strong leadership.
- Strengthen mental health nursing education.

## Compassion in practice: the Chief Nursing Officer's vision and strategy for nursing, midwifery, and care staff in England (2013)

This vision[9] identifies six qualities (six Cs) that are required of all nurses, midwives, and care staff (see Figure 1.1 and Table 1.2):
- *Care*—put care at the heart of nursing and all health and social care organizations. It is argued that care is the essence of mental health nursing. Mental health nurses can care by 'mobilizing hope, confidence and trust between themselves and the persons for whom they care'[10].
- *Compassion*—show a profound awareness and understanding of suffering and take steps to relieve it.[11]
- *Competence*—deliver effective care that is based on the best available and best possible evidence.
- *Communication*—use the most effective communication skills (➔ p. 54).
- *Courage*—have the personal strength and vision to defend and uphold the best possible care.
- *Commitment*—pledge to provide the most effective care at all times and in all circumstances.

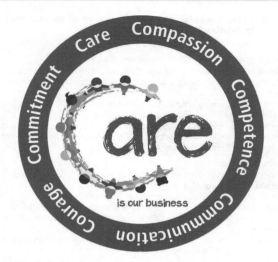

Fig. 1.1 The six Cs vision for nurses, midwives, and care staff in England. (Reproduced from NHS England ᔕ www.england.nhs.uk under the Open Government Licence.)

Table 1.2 The mental health nursing contribution to 'No Health Without Mental Health' (ᔕ www.england.nhs.uk/wp-content/uploads/2012/12/6c-mental-health.pdf)

| Levels of public mental health nursing | Role of the mental health nurse in health promotion to improve mental health and emotional well-being | Mental health nursing outcomes |
| --- | --- | --- |
| **Level 1** All mental health nurses maximize their role in health and well-being. Promote equitable care for all groups and individuals. Help to reduce stigma and discrimination | Increase resilience, promote self-esteem, life and coping skills<br>Assess, refer, and delegate to maximize resources and use expertise of others<br>Ensure preventative action and early intervention are a core component of assessment and care planning | Demonstrate improved therapeutic engagement with service users in the health and care system<br>Achieve yearly reduction in the numbers of cases of self-harm and suicide among psychiatric inpatients |

(continued)

**Table 1.2** (Contd)

| Levels of public mental health nursing | Role of the mental health nurse in health promotion to improve mental health and emotional well-being | Mental health nursing outcomes |
| --- | --- | --- |
| **Level 2** Mental health nurses with specific primary and secondary prevention roles such as early intervention, working with families with multiple problems and people with long-term illness and comorbidity (e.g. diabetes, depression)<br><br>**Level 3** Mental health nurses advise, support, and work in partnership with public health practitioners such as health visitors, school nurses, and occupational health nurses (e.g. anti-bullying policies) | Target particular public health needs (e.g. school-aged children, vulnerable children such as those in care)<br><br>Lead on care of people with complex and/or additional needs, including support, education, and training for families, carers, and school/care staff<br><br>Provide proactive early intervention and leadership as part of a multi-agency team, for people with multiple problems (e.g. young offenders, military veterans)<br><br>Use evidence-based approaches to deliver cost-effective programmes and interventions<br><br>Promote access and reduce barriers to mental health services, reduce stigma, discrimination, and inequalities, and promote social inclusion | Reduce the number of violent and aggressive incidents within psychiatric inpatient wards<br><br>Demonstrate a year-on-year reduction in the number of falls sustained by older people<br><br>Demonstrate improved use of observation and engagement in psychiatric inpatient wards<br><br>Demonstrate improved nutrition awareness and physical activity<br><br>Demonstrate a reduction in medication errors<br><br>Improve medication adherence |

## References

5  Department of Health. *Values into Action: the Chief Nursing Officer's Review of Mental Health Nursing in England*. Department of Health: London, 2006.
6  Department of Health. *Values into Action: the Chief Nursing Officer's Review of Mental Health Nursing in England. Best practice competencies and capabilities for mental health nursing education*. Department of Health: London, 2006.
7  Department of Health. *Values into Action: the Chief Nursing Officer's Review of Mental Health Nursing in England. Self-assessment toolkit*. Department of Health: London, 2006.
8  Scottish Government. *Rights, Relationships and Recovery: the Report of the National Review of Mental Health Nursing in Scotland*. NHS Scotland: Edinburgh, 2006. ℗ www.scotland.gov.uk/Publications/2006/04/18164814/0
9  Department of Health. *Compassion in Practice: a vision and strategy for nurses, midwives and care staff*. Department of Health: London, 2013.
10  Stickley T and Stacey G. Caring: the essence of mental health nursing. In: P Callaghan, J Playle and L Cooper (eds) *Mental Health Nursing Skills*. Oxford University Press: Oxford, 2006. pp. 44–54.
11  Gilbert P. *The Compassionate Mind*. Constable: London, 2009.

# Integrated health care

### Mental health and physical health: the issues

There is considerable overlap between mental health and physical health problems:

- Approximately 4.6 million people (30%) in the UK with a long-term physical condition have a mental health problem.
- Around 46% of people with a mental health problem have a long-term condition.[12]
- Quality-of-life scores for people with depression only are on average 72.9; for those with depression and one other physical health problem, the score drops to 58.5 depending on the condition. People with depression and two or more physical conditions have a quality-of-life score of 58.1.[13]
- There is an up to 180% increase in patient care costs for people with anxiety or depression who also have other chronic health conditions, compared with people who do not have mental health problems.[14]
- The monthly patient care costs are more than twice as high for people with mental health problems and other chronic medical conditions as they are for people with these conditions who do not have mental health problems.[12]
- People with comorbid mental and physical health problems also have poorer prognoses and self-care skills.[12]
- It is estimated that the National Health Service (NHS) spends between £8 billion and £13 billion on treating people with comorbid mental and physical health problems.[12]

### Integrating mental health and physical health assessment

An important part of addressing the integrated health care agenda is conducting assessments that incorporate mental and physical health issues. Examples of tools that can be used for this are the Wellness Recovery Action Plan (WRAP)[15] and the Three Keys Model.[16]

### The WRAP approach

WRAP[15] is based on the principle that recovery is possible. Individuals take personal responsibility for their life and well-being, working in collaboration with professionals who help them to achieve recovery, being self-aware, advocating for themselves, and enlisting the support of others.

*Components of WRAP assessment and care planning*
- The wellness toolbox—identify the tools that a person deems necessary to their health and well-being.
- Daily maintenance plan—develop a plan which will ensure that health and well-being are maintained.
- Identify triggers that enable a person to recover, as well as early warning signs of impending breakdown, and develop associated action plans that may help people to deal with these triggers.
- Crisis planning—make plans to manage a crisis.
- Post-crisis planning—make plans to avert future crises.

## The Three Keys Model

The Three Keys Model[16] promotes a shared approach to mental health assessment in which professionals work collaboratively with mental health service users. The three keys to which the model refers are summarized as follows:

- First key—active participation of the service user and carer.
- Second key—a multidisciplinary approach that is expanded to involve all agencies whom the service user identifies as relevant to their recovery.
- Third key—a focus on helping the service user to identify their strengths, needs, and 'resiliences'.

## Models of integrated care

- Pathway—this approach is characterized by developing an integrated care pathway that incorporates mental and physical health care.
- Organizational—this approach is characterized by a reorganization of services to focus on providing integrated health care.
- Information—this approach is characterized by providing information to people who are using non-integrated services on how best to access services that address other health concerns.
- Incentive—this approach incentivizes services that take an integrated approach to physical and mental health care provision.

## Evidence-based benefits associated with integrated health care

- Improved quality of life.[12]
- Reduced costs.
- More effective symptom management.
- Improved recovery.
- Better prognosis.
- Reduced hospital stays.

## Problems associated with integrated health care

- Uncertainty about what type of integration produces better outcomes.[12]
- Treatment for mental illness can increase physical health problems.
- Integration appears to involve more than simply layering services on top of one another.
- Evidence-based interventions are not always in use.

## Integrated models with promise

- Detection[12,17,18]—these are services developed to improve rates of detection of mental health problems in people with physical health problems, and vice versa. Examples include using routine mental health assessments in physical health care, and routine physical health screening in mental health care.
- Liaison mental health services in acute care—the provision of such services in acute care has been shown to have a positive effect in detecting and treating mental health problems in people with physical health problems.

- Working with the voluntary sector—multi-agency working, especially with the voluntary sector, has been shown to help people through support groups.
- Integrating mental health and primary care—increasing the provision of mental health services in primary care and seeing the latter as the focus for the delivery of mental health care.
- Self-management—using self-help groups and guided self-help approaches to enable people to manage and live better with their problems.

## Developing and evaluating integrated health care services

*Collaborative care for people with comorbid mental health problems*
The characteristics of the collaborative care approach[12,19] are as follows:
- A care manager with overall responsibility for coordinating the collaborative care approach through linking with all of the agencies necessary for the provision of a comprehensive care package.
- A structured care management plan that is developed and agreed with the service user.
- Systematic follow-up to ensure ongoing assessment and intervention where necessary.
- A multiprofessional approach with processes to ensure closer working between all those involved from primary care and mental health care.
- Service user education and support for guided self-management and care.
- A stepped care approach that starts with watchful waiting, and limits intensive care to those in most need and who are not responding to initial interventions.

*Clinical commissioning groups (CCGs)*
From 1 April 2013 the UK coalition government introduced sweeping changes to the organization of the NHS in England. Commissioning of health services is the responsibility of CCGs which consist largely of GPs and other health care professionals who determine what services are needed for the population whom they serve. CCGs have responsibility for the quality and productivity of care, and can help the integrated health care agenda by commissioning those services that have integrated health care at their heart.

*Commissioning for Quality and Innovation (CQUIN)*
CQUIN payments can provide an incentive for services to adopt an integrated approach. Services may be more likely to develop new, integrated approaches if they know that doing so will have financial benefits.

*Recommendations for services*
- Incorporate disease management and rehabilitation by including mental health services.
- Consider investing in liaison mental health services.
- Train primary care professionals in mental health skills.
- Consider using tools for integrating health care, such as WRAP.
- Target people with long-term conditions and comorbid mental health problems.
- Provide advice and interventions that prevent mental health problems from developing in people with long-term conditions.

# References

12 Naylor C et al. *Long-Term Conditions and Mental Health: the cost of co-morbidities*. The King's Fund and Centre for Mental Health: London, 2012.

13 Mousasavi S et al. Depression, chronic disease and decrements in health: results from the World Health Surveys. *The Lancet* 2007; **370**: 851–88.

14 Melek S and Norris D. *Chronic Conditions and Comorbid Psychological Disorders*. Milliman Research Report. Milliman: Seattle, 2008.

15 Wrap® and Recovery Books. ℰ www.mentalhealthrecovery.com/wrap

16 The National Institute for Mental Health in England (NIMHE) and the Care Services Improvement Partnership. *3 Keys to a Shared Approach in Mental Health Assessment*. Department of Health: London, 2008.

17 Harrison M et al. A secondary analysis of the moderating effects of depression and multimorbidity on the effectiveness of a chronic disease self-management programme. *Patient Education and Counseling* 2012; **87**: 67–73.

18 National Institute for Health and Care Excellence (NICE). *Chronic Obstructive Pulmonary Disease: management of chronic obstructive pulmonary disease in adults in primary and secondary care (partial update)*. CG101. NICE: London, 2010. ℰ www.nice.org.uk/guidance/cg101/resources/guidance-chronic-obstructive-pulmonary-disease-pdf

19 National Institute for Health and Care Excellence (NICE). *Depression in Adults with a Chronic Physical Health Problem: treatment and management*. CG91. NICE: London, 2009. ℰ www.nice.org.uk/guidance/cg91

## Co-production

Co-production has been defined as a relationship in which professionals and citizens share power to plan and deliver services, recognizing that egalitarian partnerships improve quality of life and services for people and communities.

The six principles of co-production are as follows:
- Taking an assets-based approach—people are not passive recipients but equal partners in the design and delivery of services.
- Building on people's existing capabilities—altering service models so that they provide opportunities for people's capabilities to grow.
- Reciprocity and mutuality—offering people a range of incentives to work in reciprocal relationships with professionals so that there are mutual responsibilities and expectations.
- Peer support networks—engaging personal networks alongside professional ones as the most effective way of transferring knowledge.
- Blurring distinctions between producers and consumers of services by reconfiguring the way that services are developed and delivered.
- Facilitating rather than delivering, so that public service agencies become facilitators and catalysts rather than being the main providers.

In summary, co-production includes the following elements:
- co-design, including planning of services
- co-decision making in the allocation of resources
- co-delivery of services, including the role of volunteers in providing the service
- co-evaluation of the service.[20]

In addition, the Social Care Institute for Excellence (SCIE)[21] has highlighted that co-designing services (i.e. managers and citizens working together in the planning stages of projects), although important, must be accompanied by co-delivery (i.e. involving people in actual service provision). It is therefore useful to consider co-production at different levels. For example:
- descriptive—where co-production already takes place in the delivery of services as people who use services and carers work together to achieve individual outcomes, but activities cannot challenge the way that services are delivered, and co-production is not really recognized
- intermediate—where there is more recognition and mutual respect, such as where individuals who use services are involved in the recruitment and training of professionals
- transformative—where new relationships between staff and individuals who use services are created, where people who use services are recognized as experts in their own right. There is respect for the assets that everyone brings to the process, and an emphasis on all the outcomes that people value, rather than just on those that the organization values, such as clinical outcomes.[22]

## References

20  Löffler E. A future research agenda for co-production: overview paper. In: *Local Authorities and Research Councils' Initiative. Co-production: a series of commissioned reports.* Research Councils UK: Swindon, 2010.

21  Social Care Institute for Excellence (SCIE). *Co-Production in Social Care: what it is and how to do it.* SCIE: London, 2014. ℘ www.scie.org.uk/publications/guides/guide51/what-is-coproduction/defining-coproduction.asp

22  Needham C and Carr S. *SCIE Research Briefing 31: Co-production: an emerging evidence base for adult social care transformation.* Social Care Institute for Excellence: London, 2009.

## Further reading

Stephens L, Ryan-Collins J and Boyle D. *Co-Production: a Manifesto for growing the core economy.* The New Economics Foundation: London, 2008. ℘ http://b.3cdn.net/nefoundation/5abec531b2a775dc8d_qjm6bqzpt.pdf

# Promoting recovery through therapeutic communication

## Introduction

Mental health nurses' sound interpersonal skills help people to recover from mental distress so that they can lead meaningful and satisfying lives.[23] A focus on recovery-oriented practice is a core part of 'No Health without Mental Health', the national mental health strategy.[24] There are several ways in which mental health nurses can promote people's recovery through sound interpersonal communication.

## Key interpersonal skills to promote recovery

- Listen actively to help the person to make sense of their mental health problems.[23]
- Help the person to identify and prioritize *their* personal goals for recovery.
- Demonstrate a belief in the person's existing strengths and resources in relation to their pursuit of personal goals.
- Identify examples from your own 'lived experience', or that of other service users, which inspire and validate people's goals.
- Pay particular attention to the importance of goals that take the person out of the sick role and enable them to contribute actively to the lives of others.
- Identify non-mental health resources—friends, contacts, and organizations—that are relevant to the achievement of the person's goals.
- Encourage self-management of mental health problems—by providing information, or reinforcing coping strategies.
- Discuss what kind of therapeutic interventions the person wants, and respect their wishes where possible.
- Behave at all times in such a way as to convey an attitude of respect for the person and a desire for an equal partnership in working together, indicating a willingness to go the extra mile.
- While accepting that the future is uncertain and setbacks can occur, continue to express support for the idea that it is possible to achieve these self-defined goals, thereby maintaining hope and positive expectations.

## References

23 Shepherd G, Boardman J and Slade M. *Ten Top Tips for Recovery-Oriented Practice*. Sainsbury Centre for Mental Health: London, 2009.
24 Department of Health. *No Health Without Mental Health: delivering better mental health outcomes for people of all ages*. Department of Health: London, 2011.

## Further reading

Morrissey J and Callaghan P. *Communication Skills for Mental Health Nurses*. Open University Press: Buckingham, 2011.

# Therapeutic value of phatic communication

### Introduction

Phatic communication, or 'small talk',[25] focuses less on the content of communication, and more on the mere act of communicating, such as when we greet someone with a polite 'Good morning'. Phatic communication helps us to express camaraderie with others and opens up opportunities for the more emphatic communication (i.e. communicating for a specific purpose) that characterizes much of mental health nursing.

### Using phatic communication

*Suggested topics to talk about*[26]
- The weather.
- Current affairs.
- Sports.
- Entertainment.
- Things you have in common.
- The prices in the shops.

*Topics to avoid talking about*
- Subjects that could cause offence.
- A person's earnings.
- Sensitive personal issues.
- Controversial topics.

### Phatic communication in mental health nursing: benefits and pitfalls

*Benefits*[26]
- It helps to avoid uncomfortable silences.
- It demonstrates spontaneity.
- It is intuitive (i.e. done without much thought).
- It uses the nurse's own experience.
- It is not impeded by issues of confidentiality.
- It is not forced.
- It relies little on formal skill.
- It does not require costly training or preparation.
- It is not bound by formal rules of communication.
- It breaks down professional barriers.

*Pitfalls*
- Cues that require therapeutic intervention could be missed.
- The listener may become impatient.
- There is a danger of undermining one's professional credibility.
- There can be a tendency to compete to take turns.
- There is a danger of communicating insignificance.
- Speech could appear ritualized, conventional, and pedestrian.
- It is not essential to the development of sound interpersonal skills.

## References

25 Burnard P. Ordinary chat and therapeutic conversation: phatic communication and mental health nursing. *Journal of Psychiatric and Mental Health Nursing* 2003; **10**: 678–82.
26 Morrissey J and Callaghan P. *Communication Skills for Mental Health Nurses*. Open University Press: Buckingham, 2011.

# Therapeutic use of self

## Introduction

You can use yourself therapeutically by applying personality factors and your insights, judgements, and perceptions in your everyday practice. These are often seen as common factors in the therapeutic process that can be used within any approach (see Table 1.3).

**Table 1.3** Components of the therapeutic use of self

| Component | Example |
|---|---|
| Personality, insights, perceptions, and judgements | Insight is a high degree of self-awareness |
| | Recognizing a person's individuality |
| | Using self-disclosure, expressing empathy, and unconditional positive regard |
| Self-awareness | Reflecting upon ourselves |
| | Paying attention to ourselves |
| | Identifying what it is within ourselves that we can use therapeutically |
| Self-esteem | Assessment of our self-worth |
| | Beliefs about ourselves |
| | Expressing hope, despair, and pride |
| Self-efficacy | Mastery: developing expertise in a skill and then successfully using this skill |
| | Modelling: demonstrating the successful use of the skill to others |
| | Social persuasion: encouraging or discouraging feedback from others |
| Self-confidence | Identifying our personal qualities |
| | Being assertive |
| | Making friends easily |
| | Overcoming difficulties with relative ease |

## Further reading

Morrissey J and Callaghan P. *Communication Skills for Mental Health Nurses*. Open University Press: Buckingham, 2011.

# Solution-focused communication

## Introduction

A solution-focused communication style is one that is highly structured, with a clear purpose and goals, aimed directly at helping people to identify their own solutions to what may be troubling them, and having an end point that the nurse and service user agree at the outset. A solution-focused communication style has been shown to be effective for people who are experiencing depression, eating disorders, substance misuse, or sexual abuse.

## Common questions in a solution-focused encounter

These include the following:

- What are you hoping to achieve from our discussion today? [27,28]
- What problem would you like to address today?
- How would life seem without this problem?
- Imagine that you wake up tomorrow and you have realized all your hopes. What do you think would be different?
- Think of a time when you had realized your hopes in the past. What did you do then?
- What did this feel like?
- What things would you, or people close to you, notice if you realized some of your hopes now?
- When you realized your hopes in the past, what was particularly helpful and what was challenging?
- On a scale of 1 to 10, where 1 is the lowest score and 10 is the highest, how would you rate your general problem-solving skills?
- What is your assessment of how this discussion has helped you to achieve what you had hoped to achieve?

## References

27  Iveson C. Solution-focussed brief therapy. *Advances in Psychiatric Treatment* 2002; **8**: 149–57.
28  Smith S, Adam D, Kirkpatrick P and McRobie G. Using solution-focused communication to support patients. *Nursing Standard* 2011; **25**: 42–7.

# Cooperative communication

Cooperative communication is a style that is designed to prevent conflict. Bacal[29] distinguishes between cooperative communication and conflict-provoking communication, the latter being a style that may stir up conflict.

## Examples of cooperative communication

- Listening actively.
- Expressing empathy.
- Being assertive.
- Being responsive by changing a behaviour that may be unhealthy.

## Characteristics of cooperative communication

- A focus on problem solving.
- Highlighting the present and the future.
- Using qualifiers (e.g. 'It might be', 'Perhaps').
- Admitting that you could be wrong.
- Allowing people to opt out.
- Not labelling people.

Morrissey and Callaghan[30] have shown how cooperative communication can be used to replace conflict-provoking styles (see Table 1.4).

**Table 1.4** Replacing conflict-provoking styles with cooperative communication

| | Conflict-provoking statements | Cooperative communication alternatives |
|---|---|---|
| 1 | 'You aren't listening, are you?' | 'It would help me if I could finish, then I'd like to hear your views' |
| 2 | 'We tried that before and it didn't work' | 'I remember trying this before and it didn't work for me. What might be different now that may make it worth trying again?' |
| 3 | 'It's your fault that we are in this mess' | 'This situation feels messy. What might we do to change it?' |
| 4 | 'I can't believe you're making a fuss about this' | 'I'm not sure I understand your reaction. Could you explain it a bit more?' |
| 5 | 'This is the only way to do it right' | 'Have you tried this approach? I've found it helpful in the past' |

## References

29 Bacal R. *Conflict Prevention in the Workplace: using cooperative communication.* Bacal & Associates: Winnipeg, 1998.
30 Morrissey J and Callaghan P. *Communication Skills for Mental Health Nurses.* Open University Press: Buckingham, 2011.

# Fostering compassion in mental health nursing

## Introduction

Compassion involves showing a profound awareness and understanding of suffering, and taking steps to relieve it.[31] *The NHS Constitution*[32] describes compassion as a core NHS value. Compassion is a fundamental prerequisite for nurses, and a lack of it is often cited as the main reason for the failure of nursing care.[33,34] When people receive compassion when using the NHS, they are generally satisfied with their care.

## Ways in which mental health nurses can express compassion

- Expressing empathy (➔ Empathy, p. 52)—demonstrating a deep understanding of another person's experiences, and taking their perspective without losing your own.
- Being humane, kind, and generous.
- Showing respect.
- Upholding dignity.
- Being person-centred.
- Giving comfort.
- Relieving distress and suffering.
- Responding intuitively without needing to be asked.
- Being selfless.
- Going the extra mile.
- Listening actively (➔ Engaging service users and carers, p. 48).
- Being mindful—paying attention 'in the moment' to being compassionate.

## References

31 Gilbert P. *The Compassionate Mind*. Constable: London, 2009.
32 Department of Health. *The NHS Constitution: the NHS belongs to us all*. Department of Health: London, 2013. ◈ www.dh.gov.uk/prod_consum_dh/groups/dh_digitalassets/@dh/@en/documents/digitalasset/dh_132958.pdf
33 Patients Association. *Patients Not Numbers, People Not Statistics*. Patients Association: London, 2009.
34 Francis R. *Report of the Mid Staffordshire NHS Foundation Trust Public Inquiry. Executive summary*. The Stationery Office: London, 2013.

## Further reading

Firth-Cozens J and Cornwell J. *The Point of Care: enabling compassionate care in acute hospital settings*. The King's Fund: London, 2009.

# Values and attitudes for professional practice

A value is a belief or an ideal to which an individual is committed. It is an important part of the base or foundation of a profession, and is often connected to the reasoning behind practice, procedure, and policy. Attitudes reflect the values of an individual or an organization, and can be a positive or negative response to an object, person, concept, or situation (see Table 1.4).

Values and attitudes can form the basis for a profession's philosophy, and can be organized around seven key concepts:

- *Altruism*—unselfish concern for the welfare of others.
- *Dignity*—valuing the inherent worth and uniqueness of an individual.
- *Equality*—perceiving the individual as having fundamental human rights and opportunities, and treating them with fairness and impartiality.
- *Truth*—adherence to accurate facts when working with service users, colleagues, and the public.
- *Justice*—placing value on the upholding of moral and legal principles, such as fairness, equality, truthfulness, and objectivity.
- *Freedom*—the exercise of informed choice, independence, and self-direction.
- *Prudence*—the ability to govern and discipline oneself.

Attitudes and values are learned throughout an individual's life, from friends, family members, leaders, influential people, experience, culture, race, and religion. The formation of professional values and beliefs is an important part of professional socialization, and will have an impact on professional practice. The 'Six Pillars of Character',[35] which were developed by the Josephson Institute of Ethics, identify the constructs for professional behaviour and practice (see Table 1.5).

Table 1.5 Descriptions of character attributes

| Character attributes (values and attitude) | Description (behaviour) |
|---|---|
| Trustworthiness | Do what you say you are going to do<br>A person who is trustworthy:<br>• acts with integrity<br>• is honest and does not deceive<br>• keeps their promises<br>• is consistent<br>• is loyal to those who are not present<br>• is reliable<br>• is credible<br>• has a good reputation |

*(continued)*

**Table 1.5** (Contd)

| Character attributes (values and attitude) | Description (behaviour) |
|---|---|
| Respect | Treat others the way they treat you<br>A person who is respectful:<br>• is open and tolerant of differences<br>• is considerate and courteous<br>• deals peacefully with anger, disagreements, and insults<br>• treats others the way they want to be treated |
| Responsibility | Do what you are supposed to do<br>A person who is responsible:<br>• acts with self-discipline<br>• thinks before they act<br>• understands that actions create consequences<br>• is consistent<br>• is accountable |
| Fairness | Play by the rules<br>A person who is fair:<br>• is open-minded<br>• listens to others<br>• shares information<br>• does not needlessly blame others<br>• is equitable and impartial |
| Caring | Show that you care<br>A person who cares:<br>• expresses gratitude to others<br>• forgives others<br>• helps people in need<br>• is compassionate |
| Citizenship | Do your share<br>A person who is a good citizen:<br>• cooperates<br>• stays informed<br>• is a good neighbour<br>• protects the environment<br>• obeys the law<br>• exhibits civil duty<br>• seeks the common good for most people |

## Reference

35 Josephson Institute of Ethics. *Six Pillars of Character*. Josephson Institute of Ethics: Los Angeles, CA. www.josephsoninstitute.org/sixpillars.html

## Further reading

Green C. *Critical Thinking in Nursing: case studies across the curriculum*. Prentice Hall: Upper Saddle River, NJ, 2000.

Katz JR, Carter C, Bishop J and Kravits S. *Keys to Nursing Success*. Prentice Hall: Upper Saddle River, NJ, 2003.

# Transcultural mental health nursing

Transcultural nursing is a humanistic and scientific area of study. It focuses on differences and similarities between cultures with regard to health and illness, and it aims to use knowledge of people's cultural values, beliefs, and practices to provide culturally specific or culturally congruent nursing care.

Culture refers to the norms and practices of a particular group that are learned and shared, and that guide thinking, decisions, and actions. Cultural values are an individual's desired or preferred way of acting or knowing something, sustained over a period of time, and which govern their actions or decisions.

Culturally diverse nursing care is an optimal mode of health care delivery. It refers to the variability of nursing approaches needed to provide culturally appropriate care, incorporating an individual's cultural beliefs, values, and practices.

It is relevant in the UK for the following reasons:
- Minority ethnic groups have higher reported scores for psychological distress.
- Rates of psychotic illness are twice as high in African-Caribbean people as in their white counterparts.
- People from ethnic minority groups are six times more likely to be detained under the Mental Health Act.
- Women who were born in East Africa have a 40% higher suicide rate than those born in the UK.
- Irish people have 53% higher suicide rates than people from other minority ethnic groups.

To be culturally competent, the nurse needs to understand their own and their patient's world view, but to avoid stereotyping and misapplying scientific knowledge (e.g. misinterpretation of somatic symptoms). Different cultures have different perceptions of illness and disease and their causes, and this affects their approaches to health care. Culture also influences how people seek health care and how they behave towards health care providers. How people are cared for and how they respond to this care is strongly influenced by culture. Health care providers must have the ability and knowledge to communicate with all their patients and to understand health behaviours that are influenced by culture. This ability and knowledge can reduce barriers to the delivery of health care.

There are five essential elements that contribute to an organization becoming culturally competent:
- valuing diversity
- having the capacity for cultural self-assessment
- being conscious of the dynamics that occur when cultures interact
- having a workforce that reflects the local population, to enhance cultural knowledge
- development of adaptations of service delivery that reflect an understanding of cultural diversity (e.g. female-only clinics).

Major challenges to transcultural care include the following:
- Recognizing clinical differences between people from different ethnic and cultural groups.

- The challenges of communication—working with interpreters, awareness of nuances of words in different languages.
- Ethical challenges—although Western medicine is the most dominant form of medicine worldwide, it does not have all the answers. Respect for the belief systems of different cultures, and the effects of those beliefs on well-being, are crucial.
- The effect of an authority figure is not always apparent, but many people are wary of caregivers. Some may have been victims of atrocities at the hands of authorities in their homelands.

As individuals and caregivers, nurses need to learn to ask questions sensitively and to show respect for different cultural beliefs. Even more importantly, they must listen carefully to patients.

**Further reading**

Bhugra D and Bhui K. *Textbook of Cultural Psychiatry*. Cambridge University Press: Cambridge, 2011.

# Ethics

Ethics is the general term for what is described as the science of moral-ity. Philosophically, ethical behaviour is that which is right or good. In this instance, it is behaviour that conforms to professional practice. Ethics refers to principles that define behaviour as right, good, and proper. Such princi-ples do not always indicate a single 'moral' course of action, but provide a means of evaluating and deciding among competing options.

Ethical behaviour forms the basis of mental health care. There are two main sources of ethical policy guidance for mental health practitioners:

- *Source 1*. The Code of Professional Conduct for Nurses and Midwives, published by the Nursing and Midwifery Council (NMC), is specifically for nurses.[36] The NMC has also produced the following specific guidelines for mental health :
  - guidelines for the administration of medication (2002)
  - guidelines on practitioner–patient relationships and the prevention of abuse (2002).
- *Source 2*. The Code of Practice for the Mental Health Act (2014) was designed specifically to enable those with the authority to detain people under the Act to behave in a morally and ethically responsible manner.

There are seven core values that are shared by all health care regulatory bodies that govern the ethical behaviour of practitioners:

- Respect the patient, client, or service user as an individual.
- Obtain consent before giving any treatment or care (consent is an ongoing consideration and should be sought before every intervention).
- Protect confidential information.
- Cooperate with others in teams.
- Maintain professional knowledge and competence.
- Be trustworthy.
- Act to identify and minimize risk to patients, clients, and service users.

Ethics is about translating principles into actions. Consistency between what we say we value, and what our actions say we value, is a matter of personal integrity (see Table 1.6).

Table 1.6 The process of ethical decision making

| Commitment | Consciousness | Competency |
|---|---|---|
| The desire to do the right thing regardless of emotional, material, or physical cost to self | The awareness to act consistently and apply moral convictions to daily behaviour, in keeping with professional principles | The ability to collect and evaluate information, to develop alternatives, and to see potential consequences and risks |

When making ethical decisions it is important to ask yourself the following questions:
• Does your decision conflict with any core ethical values?
• Think of someone whose moral judgement you respect. Would they make the same decision?
• How will your decision affect others?
• Are your actions legal? Have you checked this?
• Are there regulations, rules, policies, or procedures that restrict your choices or actions? Have you read them?
• Would your decision be perceived as unethical?
• How would your decision look if it were reported in the media?
• Would you be proud of your decision if your child, sibling, or parent found out about it? Would you want them to make the same decision?
• Could you honestly defend your decision?
• Will you sleep soundly tonight?

## Reference
36 Nursing and Midwifery Council. *Code of Professional Conduct*. Nursing and Midwifery Council: London, 2008. See also ✍ www.nmc.org for other guidelines.

## Further reading
Department of Health. *Good Practice in Consent*. HSC2001/023. Department of Health: London, 2001.
Jones RM. *Mental Health Act Manual*, 8th edn. Sweet & Maxwell: London, 2003.

# The sociocultural context of mental health

Sociology refers to the study of the social lives of humans, groups, and societies. It is concerned with social rules and processes that bind and separate people, not only as individuals, but also as members of associations, groups, and institutions. It is relevant to today's health care institutions, whether they are in a hospital or in a community, as it helps us to understand how we got to where we are.

Ivan Illich, a well-known author of an informal series of controversial critiques of the institutions of 'modern' culture, used the concept of 'iatrogenesis' to describe illnesses caused by medical practice.[37] This concept describes the ways in which the activities of doctors may have harmful results (e.g. the adverse effects of prescribed medication). Another theme of Illich's work is the misallocation of resources, where the highest investment is allocated to technology or high-prestige medicine, such as cardiac surgery, to the detriment of the 'Cinderella services', such as mental health and care of the elderly. Some would argue that this is still the situation in the UK today. Illich has been criticized for underestimating the advances in modern health care.

Talcott Parsons, a sociologist who attempted to integrate all of the social sciences into a science of human action, emphasized the importance of health for the smooth running of society.[38] He developed the concept of the 'sick role', involving certain rights and obligations, which should restore the sick person to health as soon as possible (see Table 1.7). There is much to consider when this is applied to mental health.

While recognizing that not all illnesses are sufficiently severe to fit into the sick role, Parsons describes ways in which society expects an ill person to behave, which can account for society's attitude to those who do not conform.

**Table 1.7** Obligations and rights associated with the 'sick role'

| Obligations | Rights |
|---|---|
| The person must wish to recover as soon as possible | The person is relieved of their usual responsibilities and tasks |
| The person must seek professional advice and follow prescribed treatment | The person is accorded sympathy and support |

## Inequalities in health

Inequalities in health were first brought into the public domain with the publication of the Black Report in 1980.[39] This showed that the lower the social class to which a person belonged, the more likely they were to become ill or die prematurely. Although the focus was not on mental health, the factors concerning physical health have a direct impact on mental health; the more economically advantaged a person is, the better their health is and the greater their life chances.

There are three broad types of inequality in mental health:

- Inequality in access to health care—for example, access of refugees to primary health care or treatment for post-traumatic stress disorder (PTSD).
- Inequality in health and health outcomes—for example, there is a 6-year difference in average life expectancy for people living in different London boroughs.
- Inequalities in the determinants of health, namely access to the means of financial reward—the better educated a person is the more likely it is that they will have a higher income and therefore better housing, diet, and so on (70% of those with a psychotic disorder are unemployed).

Different groups and categories of people have very different experiences of the determinants of health. Some of these categories are well known, such as gender, age, social class, ethnicity, and geographical area. Others are less obvious, such as disability, single parenthood, quality of schooling, age of housing, and type of road user. Inequalities can become entrenched when these categories overlap (e.g. a combination of age, ethnic group, and area). In these circumstances, there can be a snowballing effect that leads to pockets of deprivation and increased rates of mental illness, such as are seen in some deprived inner-city areas.

## References

37 Illich I. *Medical Nemesis: the exploration of health*. Calder & Boyars: London, 1957.
38 Parsons T. *The Social System*. Routledge: London, 1951.
39 The Black Report. Available at ℗ www.sochealth.co.uk

## Further reading

Wilkinson R and Pickett K. *The Spirit Level: why equality is better for everyone*. Penguin Books: London, 2010.

# Accountability

Originally accountability referred to compliance with the established norms of financial management. More recently, the meaning of accountability has broadened to include the achievement of performance targets, such as those outlined in the Strategy for Mental Health, and norms external to the organization, such as the Human Rights Act.

Within health care environments there are three clear levels of accountability.

## Personal accountability

At its most general, accountability is about an individual who is responsible for a set of activities explaining or answering for their actions. In a hierarchical environment such as the NHS, it is associated with delegated authority, and is distinct from responsibility. For example, the Chief Executive is ultimately accountable for the organization, but is not responsible for individual actions of staff or service users (this is called vicarious liability).

## Professional accountability

Here there are two strands to accountability, firstly to the service user, and secondly to colleagues. Traditionally, accountability has focused on competence, and on legal and ethical conduct as determined by professional bodies, such as the NMC or the General Medical Council (GMC). These bodies establish the content areas that determine competence, but it is not possible for them to monitor an individual's practice. Colleagues are therefore accountable for enforcing professional standards of practice. More recently, accountability to individual service users has become more prominent.

## Organizational accountability

This consists of the entire management and control of an organization, including its organizational structure, its business policy, its principles, and its guidelines, with both internal and external monitoring being mandatory. It is sometimes referred to as corporate governance or corporate accountability for clinical practice. Within health care, *clinical governance* is the major framework through which the organization is held accountable to the public and to the government. This is a systematic approach to maintaining and improving the quality of patient care. It is a multidisciplinary, multi-agency activity that covers seven domains. These domains do not exist in isolation but are networked throughout the organizations to produce a seamless service (see Figure 1.2).

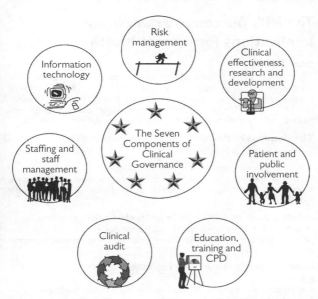

Fig. 1.2 Domains of clinical governance. CPD, continuing professional development.
🔗 www.cqc.org.uk

**Further reading**

Tiley S and Watson R. *Accountability in Nursing and Midwifery*. Wiley-Blackwell Publishing: Oxford, 2004.

# The NHS Outcomes Framework: implications for mental health

### Introduction

The NHS Outcomes Framework was designed to focus services on measuring health and social care outcomes. The purpose of the Framework is to provide a report on how well the NHS is performing, to provide accountability for how the Department of Health spends the health and social care budget, and to embed a culture of quality improvement in the NHS.[40]

### The domains of the NHS Outcomes Framework

The Framework has five domains.

*Domain 1: preventing people from dying prematurely*

Under this domain as it relates to mental health, the objective is to reduce mortality rates for people under 75 year of age with serious mental health problems.

*Domain 2: enhancing quality of life for people with long-term conditions*

Under this domain the aim is to improve the employment prospects of people with mental health problems. There is also a drive to improve diagnostic rates for dementia.

*Domain 3: helping people to recover from episodes of ill health or following injury*

This domain as it relates to mental health is focused on providing access to psychological therapies.

*Domain 4: ensuring that people have a positive experience of care*

This domain seeks to assess service users' experiences of community mental health services.

*Domain 5: treating and caring for people in a safe environment and protecting them from avoidable harm*

None of the indicators within this domain have a specific mental health focus. However, Community Treatment Orders (CTOs) under the Mental Health Act were designed to help to keep people engaged with services and to protect them from potential harm caused by losing touch with services.

### The Outcomes Framework for Scotland's Mental Health Improvement Strategy

The Scottish Government released an outcomes framework specifically for mental health in 2010.[41] The overall outcomes and the multi-agency approach for achieving them are shown in Table 1.8.

**Table 1.8** Outcomes Framework for Scotland's Mental Health Improvement Strategy

| | | | |
|---|---|---|---|
| Long-term outcomes | Increased quality of life, improved healthy life expectancy, improved mental well-being, decreased mental health problems | | |
| Intermediate outcomes | Improved physical health | | |
| Short-term outcomes | Increased physical activity | Increased physical activity | Increased knowledge about the harms of smoking. Decreased smoking |
| Reach | People at risk of mental health problems | People at risk of mental health problems | People with mental health problems |
| Outputs | Number of people taking up service | Number of people attending service | Number of people attending cessation clinics |
| Activities | Activities to promote physical activity | | Activities to promote smoking cessation |
| Inputs | Third sector | Local authority | NHS |

## References

40  Department of Health. *The NHS Outcomes Framework*. Department of Health: London, 2013. ℘ www.gov.uk/government/uploads/system/uploads/attachment_data/file/127106/121109-NHS-Outcomes-Framework-2013-14.pdf
41  NHS Health Scotland. *Outcomes Framework for Scotland's Mental Health Improvement Strategy*. NHS Health Scotland: Edinburgh, 2010.

# Recovery and rehabilitation

### Rational recovery (RR)

This involves guidance and direct instruction on self-recovery from addiction to alcohol and other drugs through planned, permanent abstinence designed as an alternative to the Alcoholics Anonymous (AA) 12-step programme (described in the next subsection). The RR programme is based on CBT and dissociation from addictive impulses via a website, books, videos, and lectures.

- RR does not regard alcoholism as a disease, but rather as a voluntary behaviour.
- RR discourages adoption of the forever 'recovering' drunk persona.
- There are no RR groups.
- Great emphasis is placed on self-efficacy.
- There are no discrete steps and no consideration of religious matters.

### The 12 steps of Alcoholics Anonymous (AA)

The primary belief of members is that their success is based on abandoning the use of self-reliance and willpower, and instead relying on God, or a 'Higher Power.'

- Step 1. Admit we were powerless over alcohol—that our lives have become unmanageable.
- Step 2. Come to believe that a power greater than ourselves could restore sanity.
- Step 3. Make a decision to turn our will and our lives over to the care of God as we understand Him.
- Step 4. Make a searching and fearless moral inventory of ourselves.
- Step 5. Admit to God, to ourselves, and to another human being the exact nature of our wrongs.
- Step 6. Be entirely ready to have God remove all our defects of character.
- Step 7. Humbly ask God to remove our shortcomings.
- Step 8. Make a list of all persons we have harmed, and be willing to make amends to them.
- Step 9. Make direct amends to such people wherever possible, except when to do so would injure them or others.
- Step 10. Continue to take personal inventory, and when we are wrong promptly admit it.
- Step 11. Seek through prayer and meditation to improve our conscious contact with God, as we understand Him.
- Step 12. Having had a spiritual awakening this message is carried to alcoholics and the principles practised in all their affairs.

(Source: Alcoholics Anonymous)

However, critics of these programmes often hold that this reliance is ineffective, and offensive or inapplicable to atheists and others who do not believe in a God.

# Essential mental health nursing skills

# Mental health assessment

Assessment is an important stage in the nursing care of people with mental health problems. It involves collecting information and using it to form a baseline to measure change and decide on the nature of any subsequent mental health care. Assessing people's mental state involves judging their psychological and physical health; this requires experience, a degree of intelligence, self-insight, social skills, objectivity, and the ability to deal with cognitive complexities. A mental health nursing assessment is often undertaken during an assessment interview, but may be an ongoing dynamic process.

Reasons for doing a mental health assessment include the following:
- to listen to a person's narrative
- to identify a person's needs and their social support networks
- to assist in developing and using appropriate interventions
- to contribute to diagnostic accuracy
- to define goals and problem solve.

## Characteristics of effective assessors

These include the following:
- experience of conducting assessments
- empathy
- general intelligence level
- ability to solve complex problems
- self-awareness and insight
- sound interpersonal skills
- ability to be objective and detached
- ability to provide a good explanation of the purpose of assessment
- ability to explain the relevance of the questions
- ability to identify strengths, resilience, and aspirations.

## What should be assessed?

- The biological self (➔ Physical health assessment, p. 38)—including body mass index (BMI) and urinalysis.
- The behavioural self—how the person thinks, feels, and acts.
- The social self—how the person interacts with others, and family history.
- The spiritual self—the person's hopes, dreams, and beliefs.
- The cultural self—the person's beliefs and morals.
- Past history—of psychiatric disorder and physical health status.
- Current financial, social functioning, and environmental factors—for example, employment, benefits, living arrangements, and social activities.
- Past and present psychiatric diagnosis and symptoms.
- Appearance and behaviour—physical appearance and reaction to situations.
- Mood—current mood and recent changes in mood.
- Speech—rate, form, volume, and quantity of information, and content.
- Form of thought—amount and rate of thought, and continuity of ideas.
- Thought content—including delusions and suicidal thoughts.
- Perception—including hallucinations and other perceptual disturbances.
- Cognition—level of consciousness, memory, orientation, concentration, and abstract thoughts.

- Insight—understanding of condition.
- Sexual health—sexual activity and contraceptive use.
- Substance use.

➔ Mental health and well-being in the global context, p. 2.

The Three Keys Approach to assessment (⌾ http://www2.warwick.ac.uk/fac/med/study/research/vbp/resources/three_keys_to_a_shared_approach.pdf) includes the following:

- active participation of the service user
- enhanced multidisciplinary and other involvement
- assessment of strengths, resilience, and aspirations.

*Using Simon's circles to assist assessment*
- Level 1: name of the person being assessed.
- Level 2: issues that the person identifies.
- Level 3: identification of current coping mechanisms.
- Level 4: record of current state in the person's own words.
- Level 5: identification of alternative or new coping method.

## Methods of data collection during assessment

*Interviews*
Interviews involve gathering information through questioning. The goal of the interview is to describe, diagnose, and begin the therapeutic relationship. The aims of the interview are to build trust and identify needs.

*Rating scales*
These are often used with interviews, as part of a mental health assessment. Some commonly used rating scales in mental health assessment include the following:
- General Health Questionnaire (GHQ)—a screening instrument designed to detect psychiatric disorders.
- Short Form-12 (SF-12)—a measure of general mental and physical health.
- Health of the Nation Outcome Scale (HoNOS)—a measure of 12 categories of behaviour and mental state linked to mental health status.
- Brief Psychiatric Rating Scale (BPRS)—a measure of psychiatric symptoms.
- Beck Depression Inventory (BDI)—a measure of depressive symptoms.
- Side Effects Checklist (SEC)—a measure of the side effects of drugs commonly used in psychiatry.
- Suicide Assessment and Management (SAM)—a measure of suicidal intent and previous self-harming behaviour.
- Social Functioning Scale (SFS)—a measure of day-to-day functioning that can be impaired by mental health problems.
- Carers' Assessment of Managing Index (CAMI)—a measure of stress and coping in people who are caring for those with mental health problems.
- Wellness Recovery Action Plan (WRAP)—a tool to support wellness and the development of self-management plans.

➔ Using rating scales, p. 74.

## Further reading

Gamble C and Brennan G (eds). *Working with Serious Mental Illness: a manual for clinical practice*, 2nd edn. Elsevier: London, 2006.

Norman I and Ryrie I (eds). *The Art and Science of Mental Health Nursing*, 2nd edn. Open University Press: Buckingham, 2013.

# Physical health assessment

The assessment of a patient's physical health is important because some mental health interventions, such as drug treatment, may cause physical side effects. People with mental health problems often have an increased risk of physical health problems, and these can exacerbate their mental health problems. Assessment of physical health provides a baseline indicator against which future changes in health can be assessed.

## Types of assessment

*Mini assessment*

This is an overview of the patient's physical health, focusing on airway, breathing, circulation, appearance, level of consciousness, and vital signs. Any recent contact with other health care professionals is also noted.

*Comprehensive assessment*

This is a detailed assessment of a patient's physical health, risk factors, and medical history.

*Focused assessment*

This is an assessment of a specific condition or problem, or an assessment of care (e.g. a neurological assessment).

*Ongoing assessment*

This is the continuous assessment of the patient's physical health status by means of regular observation and monitoring.

## What is assessed?

During a routine physical health assessment the following factors are assessed:

- *Temperature*—a Tempa-Dot™ is used. Allow 1 minute for oral measurement, or 3 minutes for axillary measurement. Alternatively, a tympanic thermometer (an electronic handheld device for measuring the body temperature through the ear, usually recorded after a few seconds) can be used. The use of mercury thermometers is not recommended as they are a potential hazard for cross-infection and risk management.
- *Pulse*—the number of beats per minute, the rhythm (regular or irregular), and the volume (how strong the pulse feels) are checked. The pulse can be felt in any artery that passes over the surface of a bone (e.g. radial, femoral, or carotid artery).
- *Respiration*—the respiratory rate and sounds are checked.
- *Blood pressure*—this measurement is vital to ensure the patient's safety. Blood pressure is measured by means of a sphygmomanometer and has two values—systolic (when the heart muscle contracts) and diastolic (when the heart muscle relaxes). The normal range for adults is 100/60–150/90 mmHg, depending on age. Blood pressure varies with age in children.
- *Mobility*—the patient's ability to move freely.
- *Nutrition*—food and fluid intake, dietary habits, and electrolyte balance.

- *Weight and height*—exact measures, body mass index (BMI), and measurements against standards for gender and ethnic group.
- *Personal hygiene*—the ability to maintain personal hygiene.
- *Elimination*—the frequency and nature of bowel and bladder movements.
- *Skin integrity*—check for bruises, cuts, appearance and elasticity of skin, risk of pressure ulcers, and oedema.
- *Sexual health*—sexual activity, contraceptive use, cervical screening or testicular examination, and HIV status.
- *Oral hygiene*—halitosis (unpleasant odour on the breath), general state of the teeth, gums, and mouth.

*Self-care ability*
- *Safety*—risk of falls, self-neglect, harm from others, or self-harm.
- *Drug and alcohol use*—substance use, and number of units of alcohol consumed per week.
- *Health-related behaviours*—for example, exercise, smoking.
- *Sleep pattern*—nature and frequency of sleep.

## Examples of physical health assessment tools
- Physical Health Check (PHC)—a tool to identify unmet physical health needs.
- McMaster Health Index.
- Piper Fatigue Scale.

## Further reading
Nash M. *Physical Health and Well-Being in Mental Health*, 2nd edn. Open University Press: Maidenhead, 2014.

# Care planning

Following an accurate assessment, the next stage in the care process is care planning. The needs that are identified during the assessment stage form the basis of the care plan. A care plan is a written account of how a person's needs may be met. A well-designed care plan should involve working in partnership with the person, and others where appropriate, and with the person's consent agreeing goals and identifying the actions necessary to achieve these goals. Three elements are useful in our approach to care planning, namely person-centred care, shared decision making, and empowering the service user. Good care planning should:

- engage the service user
- explain the purpose and procedure
- involve the service user, and others where appropriate
- *assess* (see previous topic)
- *plan* agreed goals and actions to meet these goals
- *implement* the actions
- *review* at regular intervals.

A good care plan should provide a rationale for the agreed action, and outline criteria against which to measure progress towards the agreed goals.

Table 2.1 shows an example of an agreed goal, with an action designed to achieve the goal, and a proposed review of progress, for David, a fictional character based on a real clinical example. He has recently been unable to attend work because he is unhappy, he prefers to stay in bed for most of the day, and he is neglecting his personal hygiene. As a result he is very distressed.

The long-term goal is for David to return to full-time work within 6 months.

**Table 2.1** Example of an agreed care plan

| Need | Objective | Action | Rationale | Review |
|------|-----------|--------|-----------|--------|
| David wants to be able to get out of bed each day and have a shower | David will be able to get out of bed each day for 5 days, and take a shower | David will set his alarm for 9 a.m. each day | By setting the alarm, David will be reminded of his objective to get out of bed and take a shower | By the end of 5 days David will have got out of bed each day and taken a shower |

## Tips for care planning

- Work in partnership with the service user, and where possible support them in writing the care plan.
- Use non-judgemental, user-friendly language.
- Use statements that are meaningful.
- Set agreed, measurable and aspirational goals.
- Always indicate a date for review.
- Make it clear exactly what actions are required and by whom.

## Assessing the quality of nursing care plans: the Evaluation of Nursing Documentation Schedule (ENDS)[1]

The ENDS is designed to assess the quality of nursing care plans. It has five sections pertaining to different parts of the care plan—Assessment, Planning, Problem Identification and Objective Setting, Evaluation, and Discharge Planning. There are 40 questions in total, the answers to which determine an overall score indicating the quality of the care plan.

## Reference

1 Thomas BL. *The Improvement of Care Planning Documentation in Acute Psychiatric Care.* Unpublished PhD Thesis, University of London: London, 2003.

## Further reading

Gega L. Problems, goals and care planning. In: I Norman and I Ryrie (eds) *The Art and Science of Mental Health Nursing: a textbook of principles and practice.* Open University Press: Buckingham, 2013. pp. 665–78.

# Psychosocial interventions with individuals

Psychosocial interventions (PSI) have been developed for people with serious mental illness. They are offered as part of a comprehensive care package that usually includes medication.

### Definition

The term 'psychosocial intervention' describes a number of interventions for psychosis that are based on psychological principles, but which also address the individual's social context. These include evidence-based interventions such as assessment, psychological management of symptoms, and medication management.

### Aim

The overall aim is to reduce the distress associated with symptoms by improving the person's ability to cope, and thereby promoting recovery.

### Models

Two key models inform PSI:
• The *stress-vulnerability model of psychosis* describes how stress affects psychotic symptoms.
• The *cognitive behavioural model* informs the psychological management of symptoms.

### Engagement and assessment

*Engagement* is the process of developing a working relationship by addressing issues that the patient identifies as important.

*Assessment* focuses on strengths as well as problems, and uses these to develop coping strategies and interventions.

Validated assessment tools are used to assess areas such as mental state, psychotic symptoms, social functioning, and the side effects of medication. The identification of symptoms such as anxiety or depression will need further assessment.

### Formulation

Formulation considers the relationship between symptoms and problems—for example, whether anxiety is the result of hearing voices, or whether feeling anxious leads to hearing voices.

The relationship between experiences is not always clear, and it is important not to rush the assessment stage.

### Coping strategies

Nurses can utilize a range of interventions to help people to cope with symptoms—for example, using a personal music listening device to drown out voices is a pragmatic intervention. Coping strategy enhancement is a highly structured intervention that involves a detailed analysis of the strategies that are currently being used, and replacing them or adding other strategies in a systematic manner.

## Psychoeducation

This includes exploring beliefs about the nature of schizophrenia using the stress-vulnerability model as a guide.

## Psychological management of symptoms

A form of cognitive behavioural therapy is used to modify symptoms, including hallucinations and delusions.

## Further reading

Gamble C, Ryrie I and Curthoys J. Psychosocial interventions. In: I Norman and I Ryrie (eds) *The Art and Science of Mental Health Nursing: a textbook of principles and practice.* Open University Press: Buckingham, 2013. pp. 298–325.

# Psychosocial interventions with families

Family interventions were developed for work with the families of people with schizophrenia. A significant body of evidence supporting this work has been developed over the last 50 years, although some services have been slow to offer family interventions.

Families play an important role in supporting and caring for people who are experiencing psychosis. Often they do this with little or no support from professionals.

## Definitions

The term 'family' is used loosely, to refer to relatives, partners, carers, or any other individuals who are significant to a person who is experiencing psychosis. In some cases this might include staff, such as hostel workers.

Family interventions include education, communication, and problem solving, and draw on behavioural and cognitive behavioural models. They aim to reduce the risk of relapse as well as to provide support to families.

## Working with families

It is recommended that two members of staff work with a family. This enables the modelling of good communication. Sessions are offered in the family home, as this makes it easier for family members to attend.

### Assessment

It is important to meet with each member of the family to discuss their understanding of the causes, symptoms, and treatment of psychosis. Some families have a limited understanding of these issues, and identifying their beliefs is an important part of the process.

### Education and information

The findings of the assessment are used to tailor specific educational sessions, so that the family is not given information with which they are already familiar. Information can be provided in the form of leaflets that the family are asked to read, and followed up by discussion.

### Communication

Good communication can help to reduce stress and improve problem solving. Ground rules are set with regard to communication within sessions—for example, that family members speak directly to each other rather than talking about each other, and take it in turns to speak. Family members are encouraged to praise and support each other, with the aim of building a more supportive emotional climate.

### Problem solving

Family workers discuss the various steps involved in a problem-solving approach, such as being specific about the problem, identifying solutions, setting goals, and reviewing the outcome.

## Further reading

Kuipers E, Leff J and Lam D. *Family Work for Schizophrenia: a practical guide*, 2nd edn. Gaskell: London, 2002.

Lobban F and Barrowclough C. *A Casebook of Family Interventions for Psychosis*. John Wiley & Sons: Chichester, 2009.

Smith G, Gregory K and Higgs A. *An Integrated Approach to Family Work for Psychosis: a manual for family workers*. Jessica Kingsley Publishers: London, 2007.

# Working in groups

The therapeutic work of mental health nurses is often undertaken in groups. The advantages of groups are that they are often time- and cost-effective, and they can provide multiple sources of feedback. This section outlines how nurses can work effectively in groups.

## Factors that influence the successful running of groups

*Trust*—people are more likely to participate in a group if they trust the group process and feel safe sharing information with other members of the group.

*Cohesion*—a group is cohesive when all of its members share a common therapeutic goal.

*Group roles*—the roles and functions of individuals within groups may be assigned or adopted by group members. These include task roles (e.g. information giver), maintenance roles (e.g. encourager, compromiser), and self-serving roles (e.g. blocker, aggressor).

*Power and influence*—this is the process whereby group members influence or are influenced by others through the exercise of power.

## The stages of forming and running a group

### Selecting members

This stage includes agreeing ground rules, a group contract, and terms of reference (e.g. goals, time, length, and frequency of meetings, location, start and end dates, addition of new members, attendance, confidentiality, member interaction outside the group, the roles of the group facilitator and participants, and, where necessary, fees and expenses).

### Facilitating the group

Skills in facilitating groups include ensuring adherence to ground rules, encouraging and enabling members' participation, fostering an atmosphere of open discussion, setting boundaries, and confronting people who may be adopting self-serving roles or acting in a manner that is harmful to the group.

### Ending the group

This involves bringing the group to a close in a manner that does not leave unresolved tensions, and being consistent about starting and ending on time.

## Factors that can inhibit the success of a group

These include the following:
- absenteeism
- incapacitating anxiety
- failure to end as agreed
- lack of containment of difficult issues
- hostility
- failure to facilitate hope

- dependence
- group members forming small cliques
- group members projecting ideas and behaviours on to others
- group members focusing on issues external to the group
- rivalry
- substance use
- self-harming behaviours
- regression (i.e. adult members behaving in a child-like manner).

## The effectiveness of groups

There is evidence from well-designed studies that group therapy leads to successful outcomes for people living with mental health problems, including depression, anorexia nervosa, schizophrenia, alcohol dependency, smoking cessation, and suicidal adolescents.

## Further reading

Clarke I and Wilson H (eds) *Cognitive Behaviour Therapy for Acute Inpatient Mental Health Units: working with clients, staff and the milieu.* Routledge: Hove, 2009.

Kneisl CR, Wilson HS and Trigoboff E. *Contemporary Psychiatric Mental Health Nursing.* Pearson Prentice Hall: Upper Saddle River, NJ, 2004. pp. 683–97.

Roth A and Fonagy P. *What Works for Whom? A critical review of psychotherapy research,* 2nd edn. The Guilford Press: New York, 2004.

# Engaging service users and carers

Mental health nurses should be working in partnership with service users and carers in the delivery of mental health nursing. The relationship between service users, carers, and practitioners is fluid—it could be one of collaboration with service users and carers, consultation with service users and carers, or a user-led approach.

## Getting users and carers involved

### Tokenism

Tokenism should be guarded against, as it is not cost-effective and it has a negative impact on individuals and their constituencies. The extent to which any initiative is felt to be tokenistic should be under continual review.

### Representation and diversity

The 'representativeness' of service users and carers is often questioned. Although absolute representativeness is not achievable (even with regard to lecturers or researchers), working solutions can be found. An important principle is to access a diverse local set of service users and their carers.

### The 'professionalized' service user

There is a risk that certain groups or individuals will be 'overused.' A useful approach is for new service users to be consistently and regularly approached and recruited.

### Approaching service users and carers

Attention should be paid to local need and the structure of individual service provision. A useful example is 'Ask the Experts', from the Community Care Needs Assessment Project (CCNAP; see ➲ Further reading, p. 49). Care needs to be taken to include groups who have previously been marginalized (e.g. by ethnicity).

### Good practice in working in partnership with service users and carers[2]

This can be summarized as follows:

- Involvement from the outset in new ventures and in changing existing services.
- Awareness of cultural issues that relate to different groups within the population.
- Addressing stigma and discrimination among members of the public and staff; clarity and honesty about what is possible, what is expected, and what is not possible.
- Ensuring that involvement is not tainted by coercion, control, or manipulation.
- Ensuring that there is a genuine willingness to instigate change.
- A range of involvement methods and opportunities to suit needs and abilities.
- The addressing of accessibility issues (practical and financial).
- Giving more control of involvement budgets to service user and carer groups.
- Support and supervision available on a regular basis for those involved.
- Support and finance to enable representativeness and accountability to wider groups.

- Capacity building for service users, families, and members of the public.
- Staff training in involvement in good practice.
- Involvement championed and supported from the highest levels downward.
- Support for staff to undertake involvement work.
- Clear involvement policies that are 'owned' and understood by all stakeholders.
- Monitoring and evaluation of involvement, and dissemination of results.
- Involvement being valued and being seen to be valued by service providers and planners.

## Engaging service users and carers

- *Introductions*—check the person's name, introduce yourself, and state what your role is, the aim of the interaction, and the time allotted.
- *Use non-verbal skills*—such as appropriate posture, eye contact, facial expression, and tone of voice.
- *Listen actively*—avoid interrupting, pay attention, be non-judgemental, do not give direct advice, clarify anything that is unclear, provide enough time, and do not undermine the person's problem.
- *Use verbal skills*—paraphrase (i.e. repeat back to the person in your own words what they have said), reflect on the feelings that may underpin any verbal statement, and be empathic by conveying your understanding of the impact of what the person is saying.
- *Protect confidential information*—however, be mindful that you will need to breach confidentiality if it is in the interest of the person or the public to do so, on the grounds that otherwise there is a risk of harm to the person or the public. The NMC Code of Professional Conduct (available at ✍ www.nmc-uk.org) provides guidance on this issue. For child protection issues, check the Department of Health guidelines (available at ✍ www.dh.gov.uk).

## Core attitudes and values for work with service users and carers

- Communicate respect.
- Communicate empathy.
- Communicate genuineness.

## Setting clinical boundaries

- *Behaviours*—do not give presents, make sexual contact or communicate in a sexual manner, or reveal highly personal information about yourself.
- *Language*—profanities and swearing should be avoided by both the service user and the nurse.
- *Touch*—avoid any touching beyond a handshake.

## Reference

2 Wallcraft J et al. Partnerships for better mental health worldwide: WPA recommendations on best practices in working with service users and family carers. *World Psychiatry* 2011; **10**: 229–36.

## Further reading

Community Care Needs Assessment Project (CCNAP). ✍ www.ccnap.org.uk
Simpson EL, House AO and Barkham M. *A Guide to Involving Users, Ex-Users and Carers in Mental Health Service Planning, Delivery or Research: a health technology approach.* Academic Unit of Psychiatry and Behavioural Services, University of Leeds: Leeds, 2002.

# Developing, maintaining, and ending therapeutic alliances

Mental health nursing is based on forming therapeutic relationships between nurses and service users.[3]

## Core attitudes and values for working with service users and carers

- Communicate respect.
- Communicate empathy (→ Empathy, p. 52).
- Communicate genuineness.

## Developing a therapeutic alliance

- Check the person's name and how they like to be addressed.
- Introduce yourself.
- State your role.
- State the aim of the interaction.
- State the time allotted.
- Agree ground rules for acceptable and unacceptable behaviours (see 'Setting clinical boundaries').

## Setting clinical boundaries

- *Behaviour*—do not give presents, make sexual contact or communicate in a sexual manner, or reveal highly personal information about yourself.
- *Language*— profanities and swearing should be avoided by both the service user and the nurse.
- *Touch*—avoid any touching beyond a handshake.
- *Space*—the health care setting is usually the most appropriate place to meet. If you work with the person in another setting, be mindful of safety issues, and also always remember that you are a guest.

## Maintaining the therapeutic alliance

- *Use non-verbal skills*—such as appropriate posture, eye contact, facial expression, and tone of voice.
- *Listen actively*—pay attention, avoid interrupting, be non-judgemental, do not give direct advice, clarify anything that is not clear, provide enough time, and do not undermine the person's problem.
- *Use verbal skills*—paraphrase (i.e. repeat back to the person in your own words what they have said), reflect on the feelings that may underpin any verbal statement, and be empathic by conveying your understanding of the impact of what the person is saying.
- *Protect confidential information*— however, be mindful that you will need to breach confidentiality if it is in the interest of the person or the public to do so, on the grounds that otherwise there is a risk of harm to the person or the public. The NMC Code of Professional Conduct (available at ℘ www.nmc-uk.org) provides guidance on this issue. For child protection issues, check the Department of Health guidelines (available at ℘ www.dh.gov.uk).

## Ending the therapeutic alliance

- Prepare the person for the end of the alliance.
- End the alliance in a manner that does not leave unresolved tensions or problems.
- End the alliance when the goals agreed at the beginning have been achieved.
- Leave the person feeling optimistic and hopeful.

## Reference

3 Myles P and Richards D. Clinical skills for primary care mental health practice. In: *Primary Care Mental Health* [CD-ROM 3]. Centre for Clinical and Academic Workforce Innovation, University of Lincoln: Lincoln, 2006.

## Further reading

Nursing and Midwifery Council. Too much information: what to tell and what not to tell your patients. *NMC News* 2004; July issue.

# Empathy

Empathy is a therapeutic response which demonstrates to the service user that you understand what they are going through, without needing to have gone through it yourself.[4]

Empathy involves:
- understanding the person's perception of their experiences
- accepting how the person sees him- or herself
- understanding and validating the person's experience
- examining the meaning of what the person is saying and the feelings that he or she is conveying
- communicating your understanding verbally so that the person can confirm or correct your perceptions
- communicating your sensitivity to the person's experience.

*Examples of empathic responses*

'That must have been difficult for you.'

'It seems that you found that experience quite traumatic.'

'It can't have been easy to go through that.'

## The purposes of empathy
- It demonstrates care and understanding.
- If you form any inaccurate impressions of someone, they can correct you.
- It helps to focus the discussion on what is important.
- It enables people to share their experiences with you.
- It minimizes misunderstandings, prejudice, and negative assumptions.
- It promotes therapeutic alliances.

## The five levels of empathy
- *Inaccurate reflection*—for example, conveying sympathy, being judgemental.
- *Correcting your misunderstandings*—for example, understanding the feelings associated with the person's experience.
- *Expressing your understanding by communicating empathic responses*—see 'Examples of empathic responses' earlier in this section.
- *Enhancing the person's understanding*—enabling them to improve their own awareness and insight.
- *Insight*—demonstrating a high level of insight into the meaning of the person's experiences.

## Active listening and empathy

Empathy requires the ability to actively listen.[5]
   An active listener:
- does not interrupt
- pays attention
- is non-judgemental
- does not give direct advice
- clarifies anything that is unclear
- allows adequate time
- does not undermine the person's problem.

## References

4 MentalHelp.net. ⌘ www.mentalhelp.net
5 Myles P and Richards D. Clinical skills for primary care mental health practice. In: *Primary Care Mental Health* [CD-ROM 3]. Centre for Clinical and Academic Workforce Innovation, University of Lincoln: Lincoln, 2006.

## Further reading

Morrissey J and Callaghan P. Professional helping relationships. In: *Communication Skills for Mental Health Nurses*. Open University Press: Buckingham, 2011. pp. 89–106.

# Interpersonal communication

Interpersonal communication is an interaction between people during which they convey their thoughts, feelings, emotions, and behaviour.

## The functions of interpersonal communication

Interpersonal communication is used:

- to obtain information
- to transmit information
- to develop your understanding of something
- to establish your identity or role
- to convey meaning
- to express your needs
- to control others
- for stimulation and to relieve boredom.

## Forms of interpersonal communication[6]

*Non-verbal*—this includes posture, personal space preference, eye contact, facial expression, tone of voice, and voice quality.

*Verbal*—this involves paraphrasing (i.e. repeating back to the person in your own words what they have said), reflecting on the feelings that may underpin any verbal statement, and being empathic by conveying your understanding of the impact of what the person is saying.

## Ways to improve your interpersonal communication skills

Listen actively (➲ Engaging service users and carers, p. 48):

- Convey empathy.
- Use non-verbal and verbal techniques (see earlier in this topic).
- Practise the skills.
- Solicit feedback from others.

The content shown ➲ on page 50, 'Developing, maintaining, and ending therapeutic alliances' has remained relatively unchallenged as an exemplar of effective styles of communication. However, in *Talking with Acutely Psychotic People*, Bowers and colleagues[7] describe ways in which expert mental health nurses working in acute inpatient psychiatric wards communicate with people for whom they are providing care (see Table 2.2, Figure 2.1, and Box 2.1).

**Table 2.2** Communicating with people who are having acutely psychotic experiences[7]

| | |
|---|---|
| Preparation for the interaction and its context | Setting appointments in advance |
| Moral foundations | Being hopeful, supportive, and encouraging |
| Talking about symptoms | Handling distress |
| Getting things done | Prompting people to help to solve issues of concern |
| Emotional regulation | Making positive statements and being optimistic |
| Non-verbal communication | See ➲ 'Developing, maintaining, and ending therapeutic alliances, p. 50' |
| Being with the patient | Making casual conversation and using small talk |

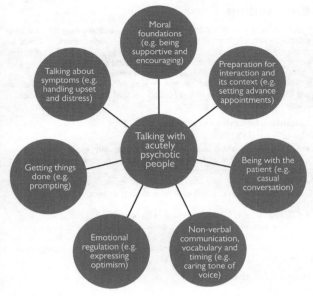

Fig. 2.1   Talking with acutely psychotic people.

---

**Box 2.1 Practice exercise: examples of communicative actions used by mental health nurses, as reported by Bowers and colleagues[7]**

- Expressing empathy.
- Communicating respect.
- A caring tone of voice.

Now give examples from what you have learned so far in this chapter of how you would apply these skills in practice.

---

### References

6  Myles P and Richards D. Clinical skills for primary care mental health practice. In: *Primary Care Mental Health* [CD-ROM 3]. Centre for Clinical and Academic Workforce Innovation, University of Lincoln: Lincoln, 2006.

7  Bowers L, Brennan G, Winship G and Theodoridou C. *Talking with Acutely Psychotic People: communication skills for nurses and others spending time with people who are very mentally ill*. City University: London, 2009.

### Further reading

Psychology Dictionary Psych Site. ℘ www.abacon.com/psychsite/dict.html

# Counselling

Counselling is a form of therapeutic communication designed to enable people to recover from distressing mental health experiences. It should be routinely considered as an option when assessing mental health problems, but is not recommended as the main intervention for severe and complex mental health problems, such as personality disorder.

There are many forms of counselling, each of which comes from a different therapeutic tradition. In this section we shall focus on cognitive behavioural and humanistic counselling.

## Cognitive behavioural therapy (CBT)

*How effective is CBT?*

- CBT has been shown to be superior to befriending, especially in the long term in people with persistent symptoms of schizophrenia, which are resistant to medication.[8]
- CBT plus standard care has been found to be more effective than standard care alone in reducing relapse rates in people living with schizophrenia.[8]
- CBT significantly benefits physical functioning in adult outpatients with chronic fatigue syndrome (CFS), when compared with relaxation or medical management.[9]
- CBT is beneficial for anxiety disorders, phobias, obsessive–compulsive disorder (OCD), chronic pain, PTSD, depression, and CFS.

## Humanistic therapy (HT)

*What is HT?*

HT is derived from humanistic psychology, the so-called third force in psychology (after psychoanalysis and behaviourism).

It is based on a set of four basic principles:

- The experiencing person is of primary interest.
- Human choice, creativity, and self-actualization are the preferred secondary topics of investigation.
- Meaningfulness must precede objectivity in the selection of research problems.
- Ultimate value is placed on the dignity of the person.

There are different forms of HT, but most of them emphasize the person's natural tendency towards growth and self-actualization. Psychological disorders arise from blocks to the person's attempts to reach their potential. These blocks may be imposed by others who want the person to lead a life directed by them. The goal of HT is to enable the person to develop their own solutions to problems (see Table 2.3).

It is believed that the main qualities of the humanistic or client-centred therapist are warmth, empathy, and genuineness. The term 'unconditional positive regard' has been used to reflect the therapist's stance.

**Table 2.3** The process of HT

| Assessment | Treatment | Evaluation |
|---|---|---|
| • Identify need/ wants of HT | • Working with awareness | • Level of awareness |
| • No diagnosis | • Carrying forward | • Goals achieved |
| • Initiate mutual decision making | • Promoting seven stages of change | • Problem-solving ability |
| • Assessment could create dichotomy | | • Level of coping |
| | | • Progress towards self-actualization |

*Indications for HT*
Like CBT, HT has been applied to a range of health problems. It is probably best suited to those who are ready and willing to engage in therapy, who are interested in their inner experience, and who have good social skills and a high need for intimacy.

*Effectiveness of HT*
• HT has been shown to be better than no treatment or waiting-list controls. The average client would move from the 50th to the 90th percentile compared with a pre-therapy sample.[10]
• HT produced more favourable outcomes in clients with relationship problems, anxiety, or depression. It produced less favourable outcomes in clients with chronic or more severe problems, such as schizophrenia.[10]

## References

8 Jones C, Cormac I, Mota J and Campbell C. Cognitive behaviour therapy for schizophrenia. *Cochrane Database of Systematic Reviews* 2004; **4**: CD000524.
9 Price JR and Couper J. Cognitive behaviour therapy for adults with chronic fatigue syndrome. *Cochrane Database of Systematic Reviews* 2008; **2**: CD001027.
10 Atkinson RL et al. *Hilgard's Introduction to Psychology*, 12th edn. Harcourt Brace: Fort Worth, TX, 2000.

## Further reading

Department of Health. *Treatment Choice in Psychological Therapies and Counselling.* Department of Health: London, 2001.
Patient.co.uk *Cognitive Behavioural Therapy (CBT).* ℘ www.patient.co.uk/health/cognitive-behavioural-therapy-cbt-leaflet

# Medication management

Medication for mental health problems should be part of a package of care. Helping service users to manage their prescribed medication is essential to ensure that the maximum benefits of treatments are realized. There is compelling evidence that psychiatric medications are effective in reducing the distress associated with symptoms, but taking medication for a sustained period is difficult for service users. About 50% of all service users will stop taking their medication in the first year, resulting in a poorer outcome.

A variety of factors influence whether or not medication is taken regularly. Service users should be helped to make informed choices about treatment. Recent National Institute for Health and Care Excellence (NICE) guidelines on medication adherence identify four key areas that need to be addressed—patient involvement in decision making, supporting adherence, reviewing medicines, and improving communication. The process of managing medication should be a collaboration between the service user and the professional, aiming to remove barriers to adherence and maximize the positive effects of treatment. Exchanging information with service users about treatment should help to enable informed choice.

A process of assessment and intervention should follow. The Chief Nursing Officer's review of mental health nursing identified four target areas for helping service users to manage their medication—symptoms, side effects, safety, and satisfaction.

## Assessment

*Symptoms*

Irrespective of the type of psychiatric medication prescribed, an assessment should be carried out to provide a baseline measurement of psychopathology. This assessment should be repeated at relevant intervals to provide a quantitative measure of change and to measure the durability of improvements. A standardized measure (e.g. the BPRS) can be used, although patient-reported outcomes using simplistic numerical scales related to improvement of target symptoms aid person-centred care.

*Side effects of medication*

All medications cause side effects, and if these are distressing the service user will find it very difficult to take the medication. An assessment of side effects is required to identify those that require intervention. Repeated measurement will identify any improvements.

*Safety*

The long-term and short-term physical safety of service users is of paramount concern. People with serious mental illness have higher rates of morbidity and mortality from physical health problems than the general population, and medication prescribed for mental health problems may exacerbate some physical illnesses. Regular comprehensive physical health screening needs to be carried out.

*Service user's views of treatment*
The service user's views about their medication will influence how they engage in treatment. An assessment of ambivalence can indicate the need for intervention (see 'Interventions', p. 59 later in this section).

## Useful assessments

These include:
- the Liverpool University Neuroleptic Side Effect Rating Scale (LUNSERS)
- the Glasgow Antipsychotic Side-effect Scale (GASS) (useful for atypical antipsychotics).

## Interventions

### Side effects

Distressing side effects should be reduced or eliminated. The appropriateness of the prescription should be evaluated in line with prescribing guidelines. Dose rescheduling to reduce the impact of side effects can be beneficial, as can practical measures, such as early exercise and healthy eating to reduce the likelihood of weight gain.

### Exploring the service user's views about treatment

Everybody feels some ambivalence about whether or not to take medication, and this uncertainty is also apparent in relation to taking psychiatric medication. The beneficial and not so beneficial aspects of taking medication can be explored with the service user. The beneficial and not so beneficial aspects of stopping the medication should also be explored. This approach helps the service user to examine their personal beliefs, and it can help to reinforce the belief that the benefits of taking medication outweigh the costs.

## Further reading

Harris N, Baker J and Gray R. *Medicines Management in Mental Health*. Wiley-Blackwell: Chichester, 2009.
National Institute for Health and Care Excellence (NICE). *Medicines Adherence: involving patients in decisions about prescribed medicines and supporting adherence*. CG76. NICE: London, 2009.
Taylor D, Paton C and Kapur S. *Prescribing guidelines in psychiatry*. The South London and Maudsley NHS Foundation Trust and Oxleas NHS Foundation Trust, 2012.

# Observations of vital signs

Patient observations are an important part of nursing care. They allow the patient's progress to be monitored, and they also ensure prompt detection of adverse events or delayed recovery. Patient observations, also known as vital signs, traditionally consist of blood pressure, temperature, pulse rate, and respiratory rate. These signs may be observed, measured, and monitored to assess an individual's level of physical functioning. Normal vital signs vary according to age, gender, weight, and exercise tolerance.

## Temperature

Temperature can be measured in many locations on the body. The mouth, ear, axilla, and rectum are the most commonly used locations. Temperature can also be measured on the forehead.

Most people think of a 'normal' body temperature as an oral temperature of 37°C. This is an average of a range of normal body temperatures. A person's actual temperature may be 0.6°C above or below 37°C. Normal body temperature changes by as much as 0.6°C throughout the day, depending on activity levels. A rectal or ear (tympanic membrane) temperature reading is 0.3–0.6°C higher than an oral temperature reading. A temperature taken in the axilla is 0.3–0.6°C lower than an oral temperature reading.

Body temperature is checked for the following reasons:

• to detect fever (above 37.8°C oral temperature reading, above 38.3°C ear or rectal temperature reading)
• to detect abnormally low body temperature (hypothermia) in people who have been exposed to cold, shock, or alcohol or drug misuse, or to detect infection in frail or elderly people
• to detect abnormally high body temperature (hyperthermia) in people who have been exposed to heat, which causes severe dehydration leading to confusion and delirium
• to help to monitor the effectiveness of a fever-reducing medication.

## Respiratory rate

The normal respiratory rate is 15–20 breaths per minute on average. Respiration will vary according to activity level, emotional state, and the use of illicit substances.

## Pulse

A normal pulse is 60–80 beats per minute (bpm) at rest. The normal pulse for an adult male is about 72 bpm. For an adult female it is 76–80 bpm, and for an elderly person it is 50–65 bpm.

## Blood pressure

Blood pressure is determined by the amount of blood that the heart pumps around the body and the amount of resistance to this blood flow in the arteries. Blood pressure normally varies during the day. It is continually changing, depending on activity, temperature, diet, emotional state, posture, physical state, and medication use.

*Blood pressure readings*

Blood pressure readings are usually given as two numbers—for example, 110 over 70 (written as 110/70) millimetres of mercury (mmHg). The first number is the systolic blood pressure reading, which represents the maximum pressure exerted when the heart muscle contracts. The second number is the diastolic blood pressure reading, which represents the pressure in the arteries when the heart muscle relaxes. The 'average' blood pressure increases from 120/70 to 150/90 mmHg with age.

*Procedure for measuring blood pressure*

- The patient should be seated, have rested for 5 minutes, and have their arm supported at heart level.
- An appropriate cuff size should be used, and the bladder should almost (at least 80%) encircle or completely encircle the arm.
- The patient should not have smoked or ingested caffeine within the previous 30 minutes.
- Measurements should be taken with a mercury sphygmomanometer, a recently calibrated aneroid manometer, or a calibrated electronic device.
- Both systolic and diastolic blood pressure should be recorded.
- Korotkoff phase V (disappearance of sound) should be used for the diastolic reading.

## Further reading

Nash M. *Physical Health and Well-Being in Mental Health Nursing: clinical skills for practice*, 2nd edn. Open University Press: Maidenhead, 2014.

# Maintaining a safe environment

People who are using mental health services should feel:

- *safe*—free from the risk of harm or abuse to self or others
- *secure*—emotionally safe and secure in that their needs are being met through therapeutic relationships
- *supported*—with access to staff who connect with them, show them genuine regard, promote their well-being, and provide sanctuary (see Table 2.4).

**Table 2.4** Essence of care benchmarks for best practice in maintaining safety

| Factor | Benchmark for best practice |
|---|---|
| Orientation to the health environment | All service users are fully orientated |
| Assessment of risk to self | All service users have a comprehensive, ongoing assessment of risk to self, with involvement of the service user and significant others |
| Assessment of risk to others | All service users have a comprehensive, ongoing assessment of risk to others, with involvement of the service user and significant others |
| Balancing observation and privacy in a safe environment | Service users are cared for in an environment that balances safe observation and privacy |
| Meeting service users' safety needs | Service users are regularly and actively involved in identifying care that meets their safety needs |
| A positive culture in which to learn from complaints and adverse incidents | There is a no-blame culture that allows a vigorous investigation of complaints, adverse incidents, and near misses, and ensures that lessons are learned and acted upon |

### The role of the mental health nurse

The mental health nurse helps to maintain a safe environment for the service user by:

- orientating the service user to the environment
- working with the service user to assess any risk to self and others
- identifying safety risks and taking immediate action to remove the cause of those risks
- setting agreed care plan goals to maintain and promote the safety and well-being of service users
- carrying out agreed interventions to ensure the safety of service users and others at all times
- reviewing the care plan at agreed intervals to ensure that goals are being met

- modifying the care plan where required, to ensure that goals are maintaining the service user's safety and well-being
- keeping accurate written records of care provided, to maintain the service user's safety and well-being.

The observation of service users on inpatient mental health units who may be at risk of harm to self or others is a key component of mental health inpatient nursing care. It is a commonly used nursing intervention for service users, and involves the allocation of one nurse (or sometimes two) to one person for a prescribed length of time, in order to provide intensive nursing care.

## Definition of observation

According to the Standing Nursing and Midwifery Advisory Committee practice guidance, 'Safe and Supportive Observation of Patients at Risk',[11] observation is defined as 'regarding the patient attentively while minimizing the extent to which they feel that they are under surveillance'.

## Purpose of observation

The main purpose of observation is to keep people safe when they are acutely mentally ill and and this experience is overwhelming and threatening to them. This is especially important for people who are assessed to be at risk of harming themselves or others, or at risk of being harmed or exploited by others.

Observation is typically used for people who are:

- suicidal or actively interested in harming themselves
- aggressive and pose a danger to others
- vulnerable
- prone to abscond
- sexually disinhibited.

## Terminology of observation

There is no universal term that is used to describe observation, but rather a number of different terms are used—for example, special, close, maximum, continuous, or constant observation, attention, or supervision, suicide watch or precaution, 15-minute or intermittent checks, specialing, one-to-one nursing, nursing observation, and formal observation.

## Conducting observation

Observation is generally carried out according to different prescribed levels, which vary in intensity according to the degree of perceived risk. Service users who are assessed as being at greatest risk of harming themselves or others are nursed on the highest level of observation, never being left alone, and the nurse is often within 'arm's reach'. The challenge for nurses who conduct observation is to maintain the safety of service users, while at the same time preserving their dignity, privacy, and autonomy.

## The decision-making process

Decisions about observation should be made jointly by the multidisciplinary team. They should be based on an assessment of risk, using an evidence-based risk assessment tool, consideration of the patient's needs, and an interview with the patient and their carer or advocate (as requested by the patient).

## Involving service users and carers in observation

Every effort should be made to involve service users and their carers and/or friends in the decision-making process, making certain that the observation procedure and the reasons for its implementation are clearly explained, and ensuring that the observation is conducted in a way that is both supportive and therapeutic.

## Safe staffing

In 2015 NHS England published a safe staffing Framework for Mental Health Wards. This framework recognizes the importance of adequate staffing levels to ensure the safety of all people on mental health wards.

## Reference

11 Department of Health. Practice guidance: safe and supportive observation of patients at risk. In: *Mental Health Nursing – Addressing Acute Concerns: Report by the Standing Nursing and Midwifery Committee.* Department of Health: London, 1999.

## Further reading

Hardcastle M, Kennard D, Grandison S and Fagin L. *Experiences of Mental Health In-patient Care: narratives from service users, carers and professionals.* Routledge: Hove, 2007.

Jones J et al. Psychiatric inpatients' experience of nursing observation: a UK perspective. *Journal of Psychosocial Nursing and Mental Health Services* 2000; **38**: 10–20.

National Patient Safety Agency. *Guidance Issued on Improving Patient Safety in Mental Health and Learning Disability Services.* National Patient Safety Agency: London, 2008. Available at ℘ www.npsa.nhs.uk/corporate/news/guidance-issued-on-improving-patient-safety-in-mental-health-and-learning-disability-services/?locale=en

# Presenting reports of work with service users at multidisciplinary meetings and case conferences

Mental health nurses are often called upon to present reports of their work with service users in multidisciplinary meetings such as ward rounds and case conferences.

## Common features of all reports

- They present facts based on evidence.
- The information that is provided can be checked and verified.
- The information should be presented in a useful manner.
- The reports are usually targeted at those with a specific interest in the topic.

## Preparing and writing reports

- Gather the information that is required in a systematic manner.
- Use information from as many sources as are necessary for a comprehensive and accurate report.
- Work in partnership with service users and their significant others when compiling the report.
- Be factual and precise.
- Avoid using abbreviations that will not be easily understood by others.
- Do not use jargon or meaningless phrases.
- Avoid irrelevant speculation.
- Avoid making offensive subjective statements.
- Write in a way that can be easily understood.
- Use evidence and/or examples to support statements or judgements.
- Use examples to clarify or illustrate the information.
- Consider the purpose of the report.
- Consider your audience.

## Presenting the report

- Be assertive.
- Speak clearly, calmly, and slowly.
- Avoid over-elaboration.
- Stick to your proposed task.
- Invite questions and comments.
- Be respectful of others.
- Stick to the time agreed.
- Make clear recommendations.
- Summarize the main points at the end.
- End with a clear take-home message.

## Further reading

www.askoxford.com

# Writing and keeping records of care

Nurses have a professional responsibility to keep accurate records of the care that they provide. The NMC acknowledges that record keeping is fundamental to nursing, and provides guidelines for nurses on records and record keeping.

## The importance of good record keeping

- Helping to improve accountability.
- Showing how decisions related to patient care were made.
- Supporting the delivery of services.
- Supporting effective clinical judgements and decisions.
- Supporting patient care and communications.
- Making continuity of care easier.
- Providing documentary evidence of services delivered to health care team.
- Helping to identify risks, and enabling early detection of complications.
- Supporting clinical audit, research, allocation of resources and performance planning.
- Helping to address complaints or legal processes.

## The content and style of records[12]

- Handwriting should be legible.
- All entries to records should be signed. In the case of written records, the person's name and job title should be printed alongside the first entry.
- In line with local policy, the date and time in real time and chronological order should be inserted on all records.
- Records must be accurate and the meaning must be clear.
- Records must be factual and free of unnecessary abbreviations, jargon, meaningless phrases or irrelevant speculation.
- Use your professional judgement to decide what is relevant to be recorded.
- Record details of any assessments and reviews, provide evidence of arrangements for future and on-going care and treatment.
- Records must identify any risks or problems and show action taken.
- You must communicate fully and effectively with colleagues, ensuring they have all the information they need about people for whom you are caring.
- You must not alter or destroy records without being authorised to do so.
- If you need to alter records, give your name and job title and sign and date the original. Alterations and the original record must be clear and auditable.
- Always, where appropriate, involve the service user and their carer in the process.
- Use easily understood language.
- Records must be readable when copied or scanned.
- Do not use coded expressions, sarcasm, or humorous abbreviations about people in your care.
- Never falsify records.

## Confidentiality

- You must be fully aware of the legal requirements and guidance regarding confidentiality and ensure your practice is in line with national and local policies.
- Familiarise yourself with the rules governing confidentiality concerning supply and use of data for secondary purposes.
- Always follow local policy and guidelines and the Research Governance Framework when using records for research purposes.
- Never discuss people in your care where you might be overhead and never leave records anywhere they might be seen by unauthorised people.
- Never take photos of any person or their family that are not clinically relevant.

## Access

- Always advise people in your care that information in their records may be seen by others involved in their care.
- Be aware of local policy in relation to people's rights to see their records.
- Uphold people's legal right to request you and others do not see their records unless withholding such information would cause serious harm to that person or others.
- Record and report to others in authority any problems accessing records or missing records.
- Never access records to find out personal information not relevant to people's care.

## Disclosure

- Unless the law or public interest requires it, never disclose information to unauthorised others without a person's explicit consent.
- You may disclose information only if it will prevent, detect, investigate or punish serious crime or prevent abuse, or serious harm to others.
- Be aware of, and know how to use information systems and tools you are required to use in practice.
- Smartcards or passwords must not be shared.
- Never leave open information systems when you have finished using them.
- Take reasonable measures to ensure your organisation's information systems are secure and use them appropriately mindful of confidentiality requirements.

## Personal and professional knowledge and skills

- You have a duty to keep up-to-date with local and national policies on information and record keeping.
- Be aware and develop your ability to communicate effectively.
- Regular auditing of your records will help you identify where improvements can be made.

## Reference

12 Nursing and Midwifery Council. *Record keeping: guidance for nurses and midwives*. Nursing and Midwifery Council: London, 2010.

## Further reading

Data Protection Act (2000).
Human Rights Act (1988).
Access to Medical Records Act (1998).
The Caldicott Committee Report Patient Identifiable Information (1997).

# Discharge planning

Discharge planning is an essential component of mental health care, and one in which nurses play an active role. The Care Programme Approach (CPA) is the basis of caring for people with mental health problems, and planning for their discharge from hospital is central to its success. Effective discharge planning is especially important for services users who are discharged on enhanced CPA.

## The role of the mental health nurse

- Build discharge planning into care plans on admission or at the earliest opportunity.
- Contribute to CPA meetings that prepare the service user and their carers for discharge.
- Work in partnership with the service user and their significant others when planning for discharge.
- Take a graded approach to discharge planning (e.g. accompanied visits to home and other facilities that the service user will participate in after discharge).
- Liaise with other members of the care team, family members, and other agencies to ensure accurate and adequate exchange of information.
- Ensure that the service user has an adequate supply of medication after discharge.
- Keep accurate written or electronic records of care provided.
- Ensure that service users and their significant others have details of who to contact in the event of problems after discharge.

## The mental health nurse as care coordinator

- Oversee care planning and resource allocation.
- Keep in close contact with the service user and their significant others.
- Advise other members of the care team about changes in the service user's circumstances that may warrant review.
- Update the service user's care plan and crisis plan.

*Requirements of the mental health nurse as care coordinator*

- Competence in delivering mental health care.
- Knowledge of the service user and their family.
- Knowledge of community services and the role of other agencies.
- Coordination skills.
- Access to resources.

## Further reading

Hall A, Kirby S and Wren M. *Care Planning in Mental Health: promoting recovery.* Blackwell Publishing: Oxford, 2008.

# Motivational interviewing

Motivational interviewing (MI) is a counselling method that is used in a range of health and social care settings and is designed to change health behaviour. It is essentially client centred, but it has a directive momentum, with the client presenting their own arguments for changing their behaviour. It is based on a collaborative alliance between the therapist and the client.[13] MI owes much to the work of Carl Rogers.[14]

## Indications for MI

MI is widely used in the treatment of problematic substance use (including smoking cessation), in treatment for lifestyle-related health problems (e.g. heart disease), and within the criminal justice system.

## The role of the therapist or counsellor in MI

The focus of MI is not on the therapist's arguments for change, but rather on the client's own agenda. The client's own motivation for changing their behaviour is developed and worked on. By avoiding arguments, expressing empathy, supporting self-efficacy, and 'rolling with resistance', an atmosphere of trust and acceptance is developed, where concerns about the behaviour can be explored.

It is important that the client is aware of the consequences of continuing the problematic behaviour. The therapist seeks to enable the client to highlight the discrepancy between what they want to achieve and their current behaviour, highlighting how changing their behaviour will help them to achieve important goals.

The belief that change is possible is an important factor, and the instillation of hope is crucial.

## Skills and techniques for MI

These include:
- skilful reflective listening
- use of open-ended and explanatory questions
- reflecting back information to the client as a statement, not a question.

## Phases of MI

- *Eliciting phase*—the therapist elicits self-motivating statements from the client.
- *Information phase*—the therapist actively seeks information from the client, and may introduce a decision matrix.
- *Negotiation phase*—the therapist must value all of the decisions that the client makes during this phase.

### Eliciting self-motivational statements

A central part of the technique involves listening for and reinforcing increases in positive expression in five key self-motivational areas:
- self-esteem
- concern about the behaviour
- competence in other areas of the client's life
- knowledge of the problem and strategies for dealing with it
- a desire for change.

## References

13 Miller WR and Rollnick S. *Motivational Interviewing: preparing people for change*. The Guilford Press: New York, 2002.
14 Rogers CR. *Client-Centred Therapy*. Houghton-Mifflin: Boston, MA, 1951.

## Further reading

Rollnick S, Miller WR and Butler CC. *Motivational Interviewing in Health Care: helping patients change behavior*. Guildford Press: New York, 2008.

## Using rating scales

A rating scale is a device for measuring a person's reported state of mind or reported behaviour, performance, attitudes, intentions, abilities, personality, beliefs, cognitive functioning or style, preferences, or coping style. The term 'rating scale' is often used synonymously with 'test', 'inventory', 'questionnaire', or 'measure'.

### The use of rating scales by mental health nurses

Rating scales can be useful in the following ways:
- They provide an assessment of a person as a baseline against which to measure the success of nursing interventions.
- They measure the behaviour of others.
- They report on aspects of people's state of mind or behaviour.
- They can be used during research as a tool to assess behaviour.
- They can be used during appraisal as an assessment of performance.

### Examples of rating scales used in mental health care

Rating scales are often used with interviews as part of a mental health assessment. Some rating scales that are commonly used in mental health care include the following:
- Positive and Negative Syndrome Scale (PANSS)—measures the positive and negative symptoms associated with schizophrenia.
- Beliefs About Voices Questionnaire (BAVQ)—assesses people's beliefs about the voices they hear.
- Self-Esteem Scale (SES)—a self-report measure of self-esteem.
- Self-Efficacy Scale—a self-report measure of confidence in one's ability to change.
- Short Form-12 (SF-12)—a measure of general mental and physical health.
- Health of the Nation Outcome Scale (HoNOS)—a measure of 12 categories of behaviour and mental state linked to mental health status.
- Brief Psychiatric Rating Scale (BPRS)—a measure of psychiatric symptoms.
- Edinburgh Postnatal Depression Scale (EPDS)—a measure of depressive symptoms associated with childbirth.
- Beck Depression Inventory (BDI)—a measure of depressive symptoms.
- Side Effects Checklist (SEC)—a measure of the side effects of drugs commonly used in psychiatry.
- Suicide Assessment and Management (SAM)—a measure of suicidal intent and previous self-harming behaviour.
- Social Functioning Scale (SFS)—a measure of day-to-day functioning that can be impaired by mental health problems.
- Carers' Assessment of Managing Index (CAMI)—a measure of stress and coping in individuals who are caring for people with mental health problems.
- Nurses' Observation Scale for Inpatient Evaluation (NOSIE)—a measure of service users' state of mind and behaviour in an inpatient mental health setting.
- Nurses' Evaluation Rating Scale (NERS)—a measure of service users' behaviour in an inpatient setting that might indicate level of dependency.

**Further reading**

Gamble C and Brennan G. Assessments: a rationale for choosing and using. In: C Gamble and G Brennan (eds) *Working with Serious Mental Illness: a manual for clinical practice*, 2nd edn. Balliere Tindall: London, 2006. pp. 111–32.

# Crisis intervention

Many people with severe mental health problems, such as schizophrenia or bipolar disorder, experience long periods of relative well-being punctuated by episodes of acute illness. Acute episodes, or crises, can be triggered by a variety of factors, including environmental stressors.

Different people experience crises in different ways, but many will feel overwhelmed and no longer able to cope. They may feel hopeless, have distressing thoughts or perceptual disturbances, and be unable to engage in everyday activities. People in crisis may also have thoughts of harming themselves or others, and be at risk of acting on these thoughts.

### Interventions and services

Community services for people in crisis have existed for many years. For example, in the UK, the Arbours Association has almost four decades of experience in running a crisis centre for people in acute distress.[15] Generally, however, until relatively recently mental health crises were seen as problems to be managed within the hospital environment. In psychiatric hospitals, nurses and other members of the interprofessional mental health team have aimed to promote service users' safety and to facilitate recovery using combinations of psychosocial and physical therapies (including medication).

Hospitals continue to play an important part in modern systems of mental health care.[16] However, in keeping with the principle of providing services in the least restrictive environment possible, mainstream alternatives to inpatient care for people in crisis have started to emerge. Following earlier developments in Continental Europe, Australia, and North America, new multidisciplinary crisis intervention and home treatment teams have now appeared in large numbers across the UK.[17,18] These aim to provide intensive, round-the-clock services, including therapeutic PSI, rapid prescription and administration of medication, risk assessment and management, and help with practical activities. A systematic review of the effectiveness of services of this type, updated in 2012, found that:

> Care based on crisis intervention principles, with or without an ongoing home care package, appears to be a viable and acceptable way of treating people with serious mental illnesses. If this approach is to be widely implemented, it would seem that more evaluative studies are needed.[19]

Good practice in relation to people known to be vulnerable to crises includes the identification of early warning signs, and the creation of crisis management plans setting out the actions to be taken in the event of acute episodes of ill health. Both the identification of early warning signs and the writing of crisis management plans should be negotiated between practitioners, service users, and their carers.

## References

15 The Arbours Association. ♒ www.arboursassociation.org
16 Thornicroft G and Tansella M. Components of a modern mental health service: a pragmatic balance of community and hospital care. *British Journal of Psychiatry* 2004; **185**: 283–90.
17 Department of Health. *The Mental Health Policy Implementation Guide*. Department of Health: London, 2001.
18 National Audit Office. *Helping People Through Mental Health Crisis: the role of crisis resolution and home treatment services*. The Stationery Office: London, 2007.
19 Irving CB, Adams CE and Rice K. Crisis intervention for people with severe mental illnesses. *Cochrane Database of Systematic Reviews* 2012; **5**: CD001087. p. 2.

# Occupational stress in the mental health workforce

Stress can be defined as:

> a condition in which there is a marked perceived discrepancy between the demands on an individual and the individual's ability to respond, the consequences of which may be detrimental to future conditions essential for bio-psycho-social equilibrium and general well-being.[20]

In the UK, an estimated half a million employees believe that they are experiencing stress, anxiety, and/or depression as a direct result of work.[21] In a national survey of stress levels among 237 mental health social workers, Evans et al. found substantial levels of stress and burnout, amounting to approximately double the levels reported for psychiatrists.[22]

Factors leading to stress and burnout included feeling undervalued at work, excessive work demands, little control over decision making, and an overall concern about the low status of the mental health social workers compared with other professional groups. Edwards et al. examined studies on burnout and stress for all members of the mental health multidisciplinary team, and 11 studies specifically on community mental health nurses. The evidence suggested that members of community mental health teams are experiencing increasing levels of stress and burnout.[23]

The major stress factors for community mental health nurses are:

- job-based stressors—increases in workload and administration, time management problems, inappropriate referrals, and violent and suicidal patients
- role-based stressors—role conflict, responsibility and role change, and lack of time for personal study
- stressors relating to organizational structure and climate, such as NHS and legislative reforms
- stressors relating to relationships with others, such as inadequate supervision and dysfunctional community mental health teams.

There is a growing body of evidence to suggest that mental health workers experience considerable stress in the course of carrying out their work. The stress and burnout affect not only their level of performance and the success of their interventions, but also their job satisfaction and ultimately their own health.[24] Structural costs in terms of absenteeism, loss of productivity, and use of health service resources are inevitable consequences.

## References

20 Rabin S, Feldman D and Kaplan Z. Stress and intervention strategies in mental health professionals. *British Journal of Medical Psychology* 1999; **72**: 159–69.

21 Mental Health Foundation. *The Fundamental Facts*. Mental Health Foundation: London, 1999.

22 Evans S et al. Mental health, burnout and job satisfaction among mental health social workers in England and Wales. *British Journal of Psychiatry* 2006; **188**: 75–80.

23 Edwards D et al. Stress and burnout in community mental health nursing: a review of the literature. *Journal of Psychiatric and Mental Health Nursing* 2000; **7**: 7–14.

24 Carson J et al. Coping skills in mental health nursing: do they make a difference? *International Journal of Social Psychiatry* 1996; **42**: 102–11.

# Chapter 3

# Working with specific issues and concerns

# Homeless people with a mental health problem

Mental illness in homeless people may present in the form of schizophrenia, depression and other affective disorders, psychoses (including drug-induced psychosis), anxiety states, or personality disorder. Mental illness is the entry into homelessness for some people. Approximately 20% of homeless people with mental ill health are also diagnosed with substance dependence. Less than one-third of homeless people with mental illness actually receive treatment.

Homelessness and extreme poverty are distant realities for many of us. Our brief encounters with homeless people reinforce prejudices and perceptions that influence our practice as health care professionals. Without prejudices we are better health care providers, so it is essential to understand both the circumstances that lead to homelessness and the consequences of living on the street or in shelters.

## Causes of homelessness

These can include:
- lack of affordable housing
- poverty
- substance misuse and lack of appropriate services
- mental illness
- domestic violence, and abuse in the home
- relationship breakdown (partners and children)
- prison release
- changes or cuts in public services.

## Consequences of homelessness

These can include:
- coronary heart disease—a major cause of death in the homeless (up to three times higher than in the general population), due to smoking and substance abuse, nutritional inadequacies, and undertreated comorbidities.
- suicide—a higher than average risk among the homeless
- respiratory complaints—very common in inner-city populations (e.g. asthma or chronic lung disease due to the high prevalence of smoking); compromised pulmonary status, coupled with the risks associated with homelessness, increases the probability of infection
- HIV and AIDS—may result in job loss, with subsequent difficulty in establishing eligibility for disability benefits, and the effects of the social stigma of the disease
- gastrointestinal conditions—those of concern include liver disease, and peptic ulcers due to the high rate of smoking
- family planning, pregnancy, and childcare issues, particularly for homeless women
- dermatological disorders—skin diseases such as psoriasis, eczema, and dermatitis can be neglected until they become disabling

- deterioration of existing mental health problems, and the development of other mental health problems.

Homelessness can be regarded as a continuum, with rooflessness at one end and secure accommodation at the other. In between are varying degrees of fragile and insecure arrangements, such as a friend's floor or a night shelter, which leave people vulnerable to psychological stressors.

Working with the homeless requires:
- accurate diagnosis—they may have complex presentations and histories
- recognition of comorbidity
- awareness of social exclusion and contributing factors—not having an address means that they are unable to register with a doctor
- active case management at an inter-agency level
- assertive community treatment programmes that integrate mental health and social care
- street outreach programmes
- accurate risk assessment and risk management.

The following measures are helpful for homeless people with mental health problems:[1]
- concordance with prescribed medication
- minimizing stress
- avoiding alcohol and substance misuse where possible
- adequate sleep
- a healthy diet and regular exercise
- regular social contact and positive relationships
- employment
- adequate finances and housing
- engagement with a community mental health team (CMHT).

## Reference
1 Melvin P. *Mental Health and Homelessness: guidance for practitioners.* Opening Doors Project Guidance. The Queen's Nursing Institute: London, 2012. p. 5.

## Further reading
Bhugra D. *Homelessness and Mental Health: studies in social and community psychiatry.* Cambridge University Press: Cambridge, 2007.

# Women with mental health problems

## Introduction

Women are more likely than men to suffer from depression, eating disorders, and anxiety. Women often attribute their mental ill health to multiple demands (from family and work), overload (no time to relax), and isolation or lack of confidence. Women tend to focus not on personal culpability, but on the impact of the social situation (work and family, culture, religion, social class, and marital status) in which they find themselves.

Women expect services that:
- ensure safety
- promote empowerment and choice
- emphasize the underlying causes and context of women's distress
- value women's strengths, abilities, and potential for recovery.

## Suggestions for gender-sensitive practice

- Involve women in decisions about their treatment and recovery.
- Enable women to choose the gender of workers who provide physical and mental health care.
- Provide women-only spaces within the physical environment of the service.
- Address issues of importance to women at various stages of their lives, such as menstruation, parenting, menopause, physical health, side effects of medication (especially weight gain), sexual abuse, domestic violence, body image, and sexuality.
- Provide practical help with housing and financial problems, education and employment, and flexibility around childcare arrangements.
- Create opportunities for women to share with and learn from others who have had similar experiences.
- Provide women-only therapy groups, especially for issues such as domestic violence or sexual abuse.
- Advocate for women who are unable to voice their needs or stand up for themselves (e.g. in consultations where several different professionals are present).
- Collate and disseminate information about locally available resources and contacts for women.
- Acknowledge women's internal and external resources, such as personal coping strategies, strengths, and social networks.
- Attempt to understand a woman's distress in the context of her life as a whole. For example, an unresolved history of physical, sexual, or emotional abuse may be having an impact on her current mental health.
- Acknowledge that behaviours such as self-harm, disordered eating, or substance misuse may have meaning for the women concerned, and that they may need help to understand and explore this.

## Other considerations

These include:
- planning pregnancy
- the impact of pregnancy on medication concordance and mental well-being
- postpartum care for those with a known mental health problem
- child protection and safeguarding procedures
- care of the vulnerable adult
- childcare provision if an admission is pending.

## Further reading

Barnes M et al. *Women-Only and Women-Sensitive Mental Health Services: a summary report.* University of Birmingham: Birmingham, 2002.

Department of Health. *Women's Mental Health: into the mainstream.* Department of Health: London, 2002. ℳ http://webarchive.nationalarchives.gov.uk/+/www.dh.gov.uk/en/Consultations/Closedconsultations/DH_4075478

Freeman D and Freeman J. *The Stressed Sex: uncovering the truth about men, women and mental health.* Oxford University Press: Oxford, 2013.

Mental Health Foundation. *Women and Mental Health.* ℳ www.mentalhealth.org.uk/help-information/mental-health-a-z/W/women/

## People with a perceptual disorder

A perceptual disorder occurs when a person's psychological experiences cause them severe distress or severe disability. These experiences are either additional to normal experience (positive symptoms, e.g. hallucinations) or detract from normal experience (negative symptoms, e.g. social withdrawal).

### Relationship building

Basic principles of honesty and respect are the cornerstones of any trusting relationship, and this means that the clinician must be honest in terms of what they can and cannot offer. They must appreciate that the user's experiences may seem bizarre or irrational to them, but that they are real to the user, who must always be treated with consideration.

### Assessment

The aim of an assessment is to gain a shared understanding of both positive and negative symptoms. It is essential that this is carried out and recorded as a baseline for future progress to be measured against.

*Example of assessments*
- Brief Psychiatric Rating Scale (BPRS).
- Psychotic Symptom Rating Scales (PSYRATS).
- Positive and Negative Syndrome Scale (PANSS).

### Intervention

Assessment should give the lead to intervention. Service users may receive different combinations of the following, depending on the problem that causes them most distress, or that is the most debilitating.

*Psychiatric medication*
Psychiatric medication is used to balance neurotransmitters thought to influence the user's experience, including perception. Service users should be made aware of any side effects associated with their medication, and encouraged to monitor these for themselves.

*Problem- and symptom-focused psychosocial interventions (PSI)*
With PSI the service user is offered a menu of interventions to distract them from their symptoms (distraction) or to explore their symptoms and experiment with changing and controlling them (focusing).

*Social skills training*
Social skills training aims to increase the person's ability to engage in social interactions. It utilizes role play, practice, and homework in a safe environment.

*Family interventions*
These are aimed at assisting families to support the user by offering educational and problem-solving approaches.

## Evaluation

Effectiveness is evaluated by measuring the outcome of an intervention against the assessment baseline. Other issues, such as benefits, accommodation, and employment needs, should also be considered if these are identified as significant for the client.

## Further reading

Gamble C and Brennan G. *Working with Serious Mental Illness: a manual for clinical practice*, 2nd edn. London: Bailliere Tindall, 2006.

# People with a mood disorder

The term 'mood disorder' usually means depression or bipolar disorder. Biological, psychological, and social stressors increase a person's risk of developing a mood disorder. Stressors are not always identified, but include:
- physical problems, such as chronic pain or illness
- mood-altering drugs and alcohol
- loss (e.g. of relationship, sense of identity, health or choices)
- adverse life experiences leading to low self-esteem and poor coping mechanisms
- acute personal crisis
- ongoing difficulties (e.g. with relationships, school, work, or money).

Extreme or very rapid changes in mood that are causing a deteriorating quality of life, or presenting a risk to self or others, may require intervention.

## Key points for intervention
The same range of treatments should be offered to adults of all ages. Ongoing monitoring is always required.

*Mild depression*
- This is often self-limiting.
- Consider psychological treatments.

*Moderate and severe depression, psychotic depression, and bipolar disorder*
- Consider medication.
- Consider psychological treatments.

## Nursing role
*General aspects*
- Be knowledgeable, compassionate and competent in your role.
- Continually assess mood and risk.
- Establish a therapeutic alliance, with the service user as an equal partner.
- Whenever possible, involve the service user's family and friends.
- Maintain professional boundaries.
- Provide accurate information in a clear and sensitive way.

*Psychological factors*
There is a risk of reduction in motivation, self-esteem, and confidence.
- Encourage self-management—through a better understanding of the impact of triggers, their prevention, and treatment.
- Encourage anxiety management.
- Give positive reinforcement.

*Social factors*
There is a risk of social isolation.
- Collaborate with the service user on structured goal setting to encourage social activity.

*Biological factors*

There is a risk of self-neglect.

- Offer health education—provide accurate information and encourage and support improvements in:
  - sleep
  - exercise
  - diet
  - fluid intake
  - personal care
  - rest.
- Medication concordance—liaise with prescribers and provide accurate information about medication, including unwanted side effects. Discourage the use of other mood-altering substances.
- Encourage the creation of a low-stimulus environment—this is especially important for service users with elevated mood. Pay particular attention to levels of lighting, noise, activity and room temperature.

## Risks associated with working with individuals with a mood disorder

There may be increased impulsive and high-risk behaviour, including self-harm and suicide attempts. Ongoing monitoring is necessary.

- Reduce access to potentially harmful substances and situations.
- Devise a collaborative risk management plan, which should include:
  - close monitoring
  - assessment of available resources
  - risk reduction strategies
  - communication with carers
  - forming a crisis plan.

## Further reading

National Institute for Health and Care Excellence (NICE). *Depression in Adults: the treatment and management of depression in adults.* CG90. NICE: London, 2009. ℅ http://publications.nice.org.uk/depression-in-adults-cg90

Newell R and Gournay K (eds). *Mental Health Nursing: an evidence based approach.* Churchill Livingstone: London, 2000.

# People with anxiety disorders

Fear is a universal basic emotion that is not learned and which occurs across cultures. The experience of fear and anxiety is a basic survival response that helps an organism to deal with threat or danger. Fear has been described as a 'usually unpleasant response to realistic danger', whereas anxiety is 'similar to fear but without the objective source of danger'. Anxiety symptoms and disorders are prevalent and coexist within a range of mental health disorders.[1]

## Symptoms of anxiety

*Physiological symptoms*
- Cardiovascular—palpitations, heart racing.
- Respiratory—rapid breathing, shortness of breath.
- Neuromuscular—tremors, fidgeting.
- Gastrointestinal—abdominal discomfort, nausea.
- Skin—face appears flushed or pale.

*Behavioural symptoms*
- Inhibition.
- Flight (escape) or avoidance.
- Restlessness.
- Impaired coordination.

*Cognitive symptoms*
- Sensory-perceptual—hazy or foggy mind, feelings of unreality.
- Thinking difficulties—confusion, difficulty in concentrating.
- Conceptual—fear of losing control or going mad.

## Assessment and treatment questionnaires
- Problem assessment.
- Mental state examination.
- Full history assessment.
- The Fear Questionnaire.
- The Beck Anxiety Inventory and the Beck Depression Inventory.

## Main interventions

The two main interventions for anxiety disorders are exposure and cognitive behavioural therapy (CBT). There is limited evidence for the effectiveness of relaxation therapies in relieving anxiety.

*Exposure*

Exposure can be defined as 'facing something that causes fear and that has been avoided'. *In-vivo* exposure refers to exposure in real life, where the client is in the presence of the feared stimulus or situation. Imaginal exposure involves asking the client to produce an image or mental description of their feared stimuli.

When planning an exposure programme, careful assessment will reveal the range of internal and external stimuli that will reliably elicit an anxiety response. It is important that the client understands what is involved and the reasons for treatment.

*Cognitive behavioural therapy*

The focus of CBT is on the person's automatic thoughts that reflect their ongoing appraisal of events in their life. This is aided by the use of an assessment diary in which the person monitors emotional changes, thus allowing identification of the negative thoughts that preceded them. Clark has identified the following active ingredients of cognitive therapy for anxiety disorders: education, verbal discussion techniques, imagery modification, attentional manipulation, exposure to feared stimuli, manipulation of safety behaviours, and other behavioural experiments.[2]

## Stepped care

The National Institute for Health and Care Excellence (NICE) recommends a stepped care approach, consisting of the following:[3]

- Step 1: identification and assessment, education about anxiety, treatment options, and active monitoring.
- Step 2: low-intensity psychological interventions, such as individualized non-facilitated self-help, guided self-help, and psycho-educational groups.
- Step 3: high-intensity psychological intervention (CBT/applied relaxation) or a drug treatment.
- Step 4: highly specialist treatment, such as complex drug and/or psychological treatment regimens, input from multi-agency teams, crisis services, day hospitals, or inpatient care.

## References

2 Clark DA. Anxiety disorders: why they persist and how to treat them. *Behaviour Research and Therapy* 1999; **37**: S5–27.
3 National Institute for Health and Care Excellence (NICE) *Generalised anxiety disorder (with or without agoraphobia) in adults: Management of primary, secondary and community care.* London: NICE, 2016.

## Further reading

Titov N, Andrews G and McEvoy P. Using low intensity interventions in the treatment of anxiety disorders. In: J Bennett-Levy et al. (eds) *Oxford Guide to Low Intensity CBT Interventions.* Oxford University Press: Oxford, 2010. pp. 169–76.

# People with anorexia nervosa

Eight categories of eating disorder are identified in the *Diagnostic and Statistical Manual of Mental Disorders*, Fifth Edition (DSM-5). The section that follows focuses on anorexia nervosa.

## Diagnostic criteria

There are three diagnostic criteria for anorexia nervosa:
- body weight that is less than minimally normal for adults or less than minimally expected for children and adolescents
- intense fear of gaining weight or becoming fat
- body image disturbance.

## Epidemiology

The overall prevalence in the general population is probably less than 1%. Females account for 70–95% of all cases, and males account for 5–15%. Clinical samples show that the 'typical' presentation is a 15- to 25-year-old female, of higher socio-economic status. Community samples show a more equitable distribution across different socio-economic groups.

## Assessment

An assessment interview establishes the needs of the person, and agrees a therapeutic contract, if required. A brief assessment might involve determining how the person views the issue, assessing for any specific or general psychopathology, social circumstances, social functioning, and physical health status. Psychometric measures that are used in the assessment process include the Eating Attitudes Test (EAT), the Body Shape Questionnaire (BSQ), and the Setting Conditions for Anorexia Nervosa Scale (SCANS).

## NICE guidelines on the treatment and management of anorexia nervosa[4]

Recommendations from NICE include the following:
- Assessment and management should take place in a primary care setting.
- Helpful psychological interventions are cognitive analytic therapy, CBT, and interpersonal psychotherapy.
- Physical management should include managing weight gain, nutritional re-stabilization, and managing risk.

## Mental health nursing care of people with anorexia nervosa

- Assess the person's readiness to change (➲ Motivational interviewing, p. 72).
- Explore the person's perception of their illness.
- Probe for signs and symptoms that cause concern to the person and their significant others.
- Identify the advantages and drawbacks of anorexia nervosa for the person.
- Provide an alternative to unhealthy behaviours.

## Recognizing the onset of anorexia nervosa

The following *may* indicate the onset of a potential eating disorder:

- sudden changes in eating behaviour or eating pattern
- excessive interest in body shape and image
- excessive dieting behaviour, especially if the person's weight is normal
- marked changes in mood, loss of menarche, or failure to establish menarche
- severe weight loss
- emaciated appearance.

## Factors that may trigger anorexia nervosa

These include:

- taunts about body shape and weight
- acne and taunts about it
- family conflict
- family, educational, or work pressures to succeed
- other illnesses (e.g. thyroid disorders)
- growing up in a 'dieting culture'
- relationship difficulties
- reaction to loss.

## Prognosis

About 54% of people with anorexia nervosa recover. The illness has a mortality rate of 10–15%. Most deaths are caused by physical complications, and around 33% commit suicide. Predictors of an unfavourable outcome include purging, physical symptoms, advanced age at presentation, and high social status.

## Reference

4 National Institute for Health and Care Excellence (NICE). *Eating Disorders: core interventions in the treatment and management of anorexia nervosa, bulimia nervosa and related eating disorders.* CG9. NICE: London, 2004.

## Further reading

Morning D and Ross A. The person with an eating disorder. In: I Norman and I Ryrie (eds) *The Art and Science of Mental Health Nursing: a textbook of principles and practice,* 3rd edn. Open University Press: Maidenhead, 2013. pp. 587–600.

# People with bulimia nervosa

## Diagnostic criteria

According to the DSM-5 there are six diagnostic criteria for bulimia nervosa:
- episodes of compulsive binge eating
- lack of control over eating binges
- use of extreme methods to control body weight (e.g. self-induced vomiting, laxative abuse, diuretic abuse, restrictive dieting, or vigorous exercise)
- at least one binge-eating episode per week for at least 3 months
- obsessive concern with body shape, body weight, and body size
- the behaviour does not occur exclusively during episodes of anorexia nervosa.

## Epidemiology

Estimates of the overall prevalence of bulimia nervosa suggest rates of 1.3% for females and 0.1% for males. Some college studies report rates ranging from 12.5% to 18.6%.

## Assessment

An assessment interview is necessary to establish the needs of the person and agree a therapeutic contract, if required. A brief assessment might involve determining how the person views the issue, assessing for any specific or general psychopathology, social circumstances, social functioning, and physical health status. Psychometric measures used in the assessment process include the EAT and the BSQ.

## NICE guidelines on the treatment and management of bulimia nervosa[5]

Recommendations from NICE include the following:
- Helpful psychological interventions are CBT, self-help, or interpersonal psychotherapy as an alternative to CBT.
- Helpful pharmacological interventions are antidepressants such as selective serotonin reuptake inhibitors (SSRIs).
- Management of physical aspects should include assessment of fluid and electrolyte balance, plus an oral supplement if there are fluid and electrolyte imbalances.

## Mental health nursing care of people with bulimia nervosa

- Assess the person's readiness to change (➔ Motivational interviewing, p. 72).
- Explore the person's perception of their illness.
- Probe for signs and symptoms that cause concern to the person and their significant others.
- Identify the advantages and drawbacks of bulimia nervosa for the person.
- Provide an alternative to unhealthy behaviours.

## Recognizing the onset of bulimia nervosa

The following *may* indicate the onset of a potential eating disorder:

- sudden changes in eating behaviour or eating pattern
- excessive interest in body shape and image
- excessive dieting behaviour, especially when body weight is normal
- marked changes in mood, loss of menarche, or failure to establish menarche
- severe weight loss
- emaciated appearance
- excessive tooth brushing, and prolonged visits to the toilet after every meal.

Many people with bulimia experience the decay of dental enamel caused by hydrochloric acid passing through the mouth during episodes of vomiting. Frequent dental visits are often necessary.

## Factors that may trigger bulimia nervosa

These include:

- taunts about body shape and weight
- taunts about appearance (e.g. acne)
- family, educational, or work pressures to succeed
- growing up in a 'dieting culture'
- relationship difficulties
- reaction to loss.

## Prognosis

The prognosis for bulimia nervosa is generally good. Predictors of an unfavourable outcome include significant loss of self-esteem and severe personality disorder.

## Reference

5  National Institute for Health and Care Excellence (NICE) *Eating Disorders: core interventions in the treatment and management of anorexia nervosa, bulimia nervosa and related eating disorders.* CG9. NICE: London, 2004.

## Further reading

Morning D and Ross A. The person with an eating disorder. In: I Norman and I Ryrie (eds) *The Art and Science of Mental Health Nursing: a textbook of principles and practice,* 3rd edn. Open University Press: Maidenhead, 2013. pp. 587–600.

# People with substance misuse problems

### Principles of working with service users with substance misuse problems

Substance use disorders are a common and increasing social phenomenon. Substance misuse is often seen in mental health services, both as a 'primary' problem, and as a comorbidity with mental illness. Substance use problems can include the misuse of alcohol, illicit substances, and prescribed medicines.

A positive therapeutic attitude in health workers is strongly associated with better clinical outcomes in people with substance use problems.

### General principles of treatment and interventions

As previously stated, people with substance misuse disorders are a heterogeneous group, and no single treatment approach is likely to be successful for all. Often people with substance misuse problems have lengthy histories of such use before they approach services for help. Therefore even small changes in substance misuse patterns should be recognized as positive outcomes—for example, a service user who is dependent on heroin starting substitution (e.g. methadone) treatment.

### Approaches and interventions

Clinical interventions should be based on a comprehensive assessment of substance use history and current use.

Individuals with drug and alcohol problems are a very heterogeneous group, and 'treatments' and other interventions, and service contact, should match the severity of the illness or problem, and the stage of change that the person is at (see following subsections). There are a number of interventions aimed at increasing motivation to change. These include increasing awareness of the need to change, increasing concern about current use, and use as a frustration of goals. Other interventions that are useful in working with substance users include motivational interviewing and relapse prevention methods, including the use of matrices (→ Motivational interviewing, p. 72).

*The stages of change model*

This is also known as the cycle of change model,[6] and it includes the following stages: pre-contemplation, contemplation, decision, active change, maintenance, and relapse.

Most service users are at least ambivalent about their substance misuse, and this ambivalence, linked with other adverse events (such as relapses or precipitation of illness) can be used to help the service user to move further on in the cycle of change.

*Harm reduction*

Therapeutic work with service users with substance misuse problems should initially be focused on reducing substance-related harms for the person, their family, their friends, and the community. It should then go on to look at the reduction of actual substance misuse.

It is now widely recognized that the so-called 'harm reduction' approach to managing substance misuse problems is pragmatic, user focused, and meets users 'as they are', with no hard and fast rules. It acknowledges the social context of much substance misuse.

Harm reduction approaches should be viewed as being on a continuum, with abstinence at one end, and 'safer' use at the other. These approaches may use a plethora of clinical tools, including substitute prescribing, needle and syringe exchange programmes (where appropriate), drug education, and user involvement.

Substance use disorders are a major public health problem, and are also associated with a number of common social, physical, and mental health problems. Persistent or recurrent problems with substance use are categorized in the *International Classification of Diseases*, Tenth Revision (ICD-10) as either:

- *harmful use*—substance use that causes actual damage to physical or mental health for at least 1 month, or repeatedly, or
- *dependence syndrome*—a group of behavioural, physiological, and cognitive symptoms characterized by compulsion to use, impaired control of intake, withdrawal states, tolerance, and continued use, despite a subjective awareness of adverse consequences.[7]

The use of lay terms (e.g. 'drug addict', 'alcoholic', 'drug abuse') in professional health and social care settings can further stigmatize people with substance use problems, and encourages non-disclosure. It should therefore be avoided.[8]

### Substances identified in ICD-10

These include the following:
- alcohol
- opioids (including synthetic opioids and opiates)
- cannabinoids (including cannabis)
- sedative or hypnotic drugs
- cocaine
- stimulants (including amphetamines, khat, and prescribed anorectic drugs)
- hallucinogens
- tobacco
- volatile solvents
- multiple drug use (sometimes called 'polydrug use') and/or use of other substances.

### The assessment process

A comprehensive assessment of substance misuse history, current problems, and physical and psychiatric comorbidity is essential for planning effective care and support for service users, and should include the following basic elements:
- A full physical examination.
- Assessment of current substance use—use during the past month and past week. Ask the patient to describe a 'typical day' of using/drinking, from waking until the end of the day.
- Primary and/or other drug use—volume and frequency, route of administration, and use of any prescribed drugs. If any intravenous use is disclosed, consider testing the patient for viral hepatitis and other blood-borne viral illnesses.

- A urine drug screen—to confirm the history, especially where substitute prescribing is being considered.
- Past substance use history—including age at first use (and substances used), pattern of use, and progression of use.
- Social and personal circumstances—including relationships, social and support network, children at home, housing status, employment, use of leisure time, and interests.
- Reasons (motivations) for, and function of, substance use in the person's life.
- Subjective awareness of the problem. Does the patient consider their drug/alcohol use to be problematic? Have others directly influenced the patient's decision to make changes to their substance use?
- Periods of coerced or voluntary abstinence (prison, rehabilitation, or other).
- Current contact with substance misuse services.
- Current and past treatment episodes—length and type of treatment (e.g. use of harm reduction services such as needle exchanges, residential rehabilitation, community detoxification). What worked and what did not work? What were the reasons for this?
- Assessment of risk—current or past history of injecting use, HIV and hepatitis status (if known), home circumstances (children at home), safety (including risk of exploitation and sexual risk taking), and use.
- Physical and mental health—acute or long-term medical problems, including morbidity as a result of drug overdose. Current or previous mental health service contact.
- Association between use and psychiatric symptoms (e.g. exacerbation, self-medication, relapses).
- Legal and forensic issues—current or previous contact with the criminal justice system, including probation, funding of substance use, outstanding charges, type of offences (acquisitive or violent).

## References

6 Prochaska JO and Di-Clemente CC. Towards a comprehensive model of change. In: WR Miller and N Heather (eds) *Treating Addictive Behaviors: processes of change*. Plenum Press: New York, 1986. pp. 3–27.

7 World Health Organization. *Pocket Guide to the ICD-10 Classification of Mental and Behavioural Disorders*. Churchill Livingstone: Edinburgh, 1994.

8 Gerada C (ed). *RCGP Guide to the Management of Substance Misuse in Primary Care*. Royal College of General Practitioners: London, 2005.

## Further reading

Callaghan P and Jones D. Psychological interventions. In: P Phillips, O McKeown and T Sandford (eds) *Dual Diagnosis: practice in context*. Blackwell Publishing Ltd: Oxford, 2010. pp. 67–75

Department of Health. *A Summary of the Health Harms of Drugs*. Department of Health: London, 2011.

Gordon D, Burn D, Campbell A and Baker O. *The 2007 User Satisfaction Survey of Tier 2 and 3 Service Users in England*. National Treatment Agency for Substance Misuse: London, 2008.

# People with personality disorder

Personality disorder (PD) is functional impairment or psychological distress resulting from inflexible and maladaptive personality traits. The person commonly presents with problems with thinking styles, emotional regulation, and impulse control, and has particular difficulties in relating to other people. These problems are long-standing and pervasive across a variety of situations.

The main types of PD are described in the two major diagnostic classification systems—the DSM-5 and ICD-10 (see Table 3.1). Three clusters or subtypes of PD have been derived from empirical work:

- cluster A—represented by odd and eccentric behaviour
- cluster B—represented by dramatic, flamboyant, and impulsive behaviour
- cluster C—represented by anxious and fearful behaviour (see Chapter 7).

It is important to understand that each PD consists of a varied collection of impairments, and therefore different presenting problems and issues. It is rare for someone to present with one PD; comorbidity is common.

People with cluster C anxiety-based PDs most often present in primary care settings, whereas those with cluster B disorders tend to present to mental health services. PDs in cluster B have often been associated with antisocial behaviour and deliberate self-harm, leading to problems of stigmatization and social exclusion from services.[9]

Table 3.1 Classifications of personality disorders

| DSM-5 | ICD-10 |
|---|---|
| Cluster A | |
| Paranoid | Paranoid |
| Schizoid | Schizoid |
| Schizotypal | |
| Cluster B | |
| Antisocial | Dissocial |
| | Emotionally unstable |
| | (a) Impulsive type |
| Borderline | (b) Borderline type |
| Histrionic | Histrionic |
| Narcissistic | |
| Cluster C | |
| Avoidant | Anxious |
| Dependent | Dependent |
| Obsessive–compulsive | Anankastic |

A minority of people with a PD receive the treatment they need in a forensic setting, after coming into contact with the police and the courts. This has led to many people with PDs being further stigmatized as representing a danger to society. Those individuals with antisocial PD in the forensic system tend to be the ones who pose the greatest risk to others, whereas most people with PD are at greater risk of harming themselves than of harming other people.

## Key issues when working with people with PD

Working with an individual with PD is challenging for nurses, as many of the problematic behaviours are manifested in the person's interactions and relationships.

The following are important when working with people with PD:

- supervision
- effective teamwork
- emotional support
- knowledge of and empathy with the traumatic and distressing histories that are common in this group.

## Evidence-based interventions

These include:

- CBT
- cognitive analytic therapy
- dialectic behaviour therapy
- psychodynamic group therapy.

## Reference

9 Department of Health. *Personality Disorder: no longer a diagnosis of exclusion*. Department of Health: London, 2003.

## Further reading

Livesley WJ (ed.). *Handbook of Personality Disorders: theory, research and treatment*. The Guilford Press: New York, 2001.

Tennant A and Howells K. *Using Time, Not Doing Time: practitioner perspectives on personality disorder and risk*. John Wiley & Sons Ltd: Chichester, 2010.

# People who use forensic services

Forensic mental health services specialize in the assessment and treatment of people with mental health problems who are undergoing legal or court proceedings, or who have offended. People with mental health problems who have never been involved with the criminal justice system may also be treated in forensic psychiatric services if they cannot be safely managed elsewhere.

Mental health nurses provide forensic interventions in health care and penal settings, including secure hospitals, the courts, prisons, and young offenders' institutions. The level of risk posed by an individual will dictate the level of security of the setting in which they are cared for. This ranges from community services and low- or medium-secure hospitals to high-secure hospitals with dangerous and severe personality disorder (DSPD) units. Most patients in these settings are detained under the Mental Health Act 2007.

## Key skills in forensic nursing

These include:
- psychological assessment
- interpersonal and engagement skills
- inter-agency working
- risk assessment and management.

The offence for which an individual has been either charged or convicted is central to forensic nursing in any environment. Offences vary greatly, from the petty to the severe. The nurse's focus is on working with the mental health issues that led to the offending behaviour.

Nurses working in forensic services need a knowledge of therapeutic interventions, so that they can rehabilitate people with severe and enduring mental illnesses and personality-related difficulties. They also need well-developed support and supervision systems to help them to process the emotional impact of this work.

CBT-based psychotherapeutic approaches have been shown to be the most effective intervention for modifying some forms of difficult behaviour displayed by people presenting to forensic services. These treatments require time and special expertise, and are usually delivered by specialist multidisciplinary treatment teams.

People with mental health problems who have offended are often socially deprived and psychologically needy individuals who do not fit neatly into either the health service or the penal system.[10] Consequently, there is an increasing focus on developing hybrid services that combine the containment skills of the penal system with the therapeutic inputs of the health service. Nurses are key players in these developments, as the specialist nature of forensic practice is now being recognized and developed.

## Reference

10 Webb D and Harris R. *Mentally Disordered Offenders: managing people nobody owns.* Routledge: London, 1999.

## Further reading

Bowers L. *Dangerous and Severe Personality Disorder: reactions and role of the psychiatric team.* Routledge: London, 2002.

Kettles A, Woods P and Collins M. *Therapeutic Interventions for Forensic Mental Health Nurses.* Jessica Kingsley Publishers: London, 2001.

Tennant A and Howells K. *Using Time, Not Doing Time: practitioner perspectives on personality disorder and risk.* John Wiley & Sons: Chichester, 2010.

# People who are suicidal and self-harm

People with mental health problems are at greater risk of harming themselves than of harming others. The rates of self-harm have continued to rise since the 1980s, and self-harming behaviour is a particular risk factor for suicide. About 25% of all people who successfully commit suicide have attended hospital following an act of self-harm in the previous 12 months.[11]

Self-harming behaviour is commonly known as 'deliberate self-harm' (DSH). DSH involves intentional self-poisoning or self-injury, irrespective of the apparent purpose of the act.[12] The two most common types of DSH are self-poisoning (e.g. an overdose) and cutting.

## Who is at risk?

Men are three times more likely to commit suicide than women, although self-harm is more common among females, especially young women under the age of 25 years. The incidence of suicide increases with age, although there has been a recent increase in suicide among adult men under 45 years of age. Suicide and self-harm are more common in white people than in other racial or ethnic groups. Social factors such as living alone, being homeless, and being unemployed are additional risk factors.[13]

## Engagement and assessment

Self-harming patients most commonly access the health service through A&E departments, although this will depend on the nature and severity of harm caused. Successfully engaging with self-harming patients is challenging for health care professionals, as such behaviours can be difficult to comprehend, and may challenge some of our most fundamental values and beliefs.

People who self-harm have complex needs—they may have problems in their lives and feel hopeless. Any risk assessment needs to address a number of different factors and to be part of a comprehensive package of care.

## Therapeutic interventions

There are a number of strategies that can be employed to reduce self-harm or its repetition. The choice of therapeutic intervention should be based on the results of a comprehensive psychosocial assessment. For example, DSH may be related to a person's depressed mental state.

Self-harming behaviour may not only be attributed to a mental illness, but may also arise from social problems such as unemployment, debt, or problems with personal relationships.

The existing research evidence suggests that there are three useful interventions—problem-solving therapy, the use of crisis cards, and dialectical behaviour therapy.

## References

11 NHS Centre for Reviews and Dissemination. Deliberate self-harm. *Effective Health Care* 1998; 4: 1–12.
12 Hawton K and Catalan J. *Attempted Suicide: a practical guide to its nature and management.* Oxford University Press: Oxford, 1987.
13 The National Confidential Inquiry into Suicide and Homicide by People with Mental Illness, Annual Report 2014: England, Northern Ireland, Scotland and Wales. University of Manchester: Manchester, 2014.

## Further reading

Noonan I. (2009) Nursing people who self-harm or are suicidal. In: I Norman and I Ryrie (eds) *The Art and Science of Mental Health Nursing: A Textbook of Principles and Practice*, second edition. Open University Press: Maidenhead, 2009. pp. 723–46.

# Chapter 4

# Interventions

## Cognitive behavioural therapy

Cognitive behavioural therapy (CBT) is a short-term, problem-focused psychological intervention. It can be used to treat a number of psychiatric problems, including depression and anxiety. More recently, CBT has been used to reduce distress and improve functioning in more complex disorders, such as psychosis.

### The cognitive behavioural model

The underlying theoretical rationale is that how we see the world and how we feel are influenced by our thoughts. We all have typical or automatic patterns of thinking that enable us to make quick evaluations of situations. In some people, there is a bias towards a particular type of thinking, such as negative thinking in depression.

### Principles of cognitive behavioural approaches

*Collaboration*

The therapist structures the interview, but the patient identifies the problems that concern them. An inductive (or Socratic) style of questioning is used to help the patient to identify and explore their experience.

*Setting goals and measuring outcome*

Specific goals for treatment are identified. A range of tools are used to monitor outcomes, such as questionnaires, diaries, and worksheets.

*Self-help*

The patient is actively involved in monitoring their mood and their thinking. They learn how to apply the techniques, such as rating their own mood, and thereby modify their own thinking. The therapist will often set 'homework' so that the patient can continue the modification outside of the therapy session.

### Assessment

This focuses on the problems the person faces in the present, in relation to the following areas:
- life situation, relationships, and practical problems
- altered thinking
- altered emotions
- altered physical feelings or symptoms
- altered behaviour or activity levels.

### Interventions

Cognitive interventions include identifying the thoughts that had an impact on mood changing in a specific situation. A diary is used to record information and, over time, typical thinking patterns will start to emerge. Unhelpful thinking patterns are modified by techniques such as examining the evidence for the thoughts, and identifying the underlying beliefs.

Avoidance of particular activities and situations is a key feature of many problems, including anxiety and depression, and this contributes to unhelpful thinking patterns. It can be addressed by structured or graded activities.

*The effectiveness of CBT*
- No difference in overall effectiveness between CBT and other talking therapies.
- CBT was no better than other talking therapies and no better or worse in managing schizophrenia symptoms.
- CBT and other talking therapies may be better for keeping people in treatment.
- CBT is beneficial for anxiety disorders, phobias, obsessive–compulsive disorder (OCD), chronic pain, post-traumatic stress disorder (PTSD), depression, and CFS.

**Further reading**

Grant A, Mills J, Mulhern R and Short N. *Cognitive Behavioural Therapy in Mental Health Care*. Sage Publications: London, 2004.
Jones C et al. Cognitive behavioural therapy versus other psychosocial treatments for schizophrenia. *Cochrane Database of Systematic Reviews* 2012; 4: CD008712.

# Family therapy

Family therapy (or family systems therapy) is a branch of psychotherapy that treats family problems. Family therapists view the family as a system of interacting members, and therefore the problems in the family are considered to arise as an emergent property of the interactions in the system, rather than being ascribed exclusively to the 'faults' or psychological problems of individual members.

A *family* is a domestic group of people, or a number of domestic groups, typically affiliated by birth or marriage, or by comparable legal relationships including domestic partnership, adoption, or surname.

Although many people have understood familial relationships in terms of 'blood', it has been argued that the notion of 'blood' must be understood metaphorically, and that in many societies family is understood in terms of other concepts. This is especially true when considering the cultural or sexual preferences of an individual.

A family therapist usually sees several members of the family at the same time in therapy sessions. This setting has the advantage of making differences in the ways that different family members perceive mutual relations, as well as interaction patterns in the session, apparent both for the therapist and the family. These patterns frequently mirror habitual interaction patterns at home, even though the therapist is now incorporated into the family system. Therapy interventions usually focus on these patterns of interaction, rather than on analysing subconscious impulses or early childhood traumas of individuals as a Freudian therapist would do.

Depending on the circumstances, the therapist may then point out these interaction patterns, which the family might have not noticed, or suggest to individuals a different way of responding to other family members. These changes in the manner of responding may then trigger repercussions in the whole system, sometimes leading to a more satisfactory system state.

## Family work and mental illness

*Expressed emotion* is a measure of how well the relatives of a mentally ill patient express their attitude towards them when they are not present. Expressed emotion is a major factor during the recovery process of those diagnosed with psychological illnesses. The three attitudes pertaining to expressed emotion are known as hostile, critical, and emotional over-involvement.

*Hostile over-involvement*—the family members blame the patient because of their illness, believing them to be foolish and selfish, and holding them accountable for any negative action that arises.

*Critical over-involvement*—this is a combination of hostile and emotional over-involvement, where the family is in denial about any mental health problem and associated behavioural problems.

*Emotional over-involvement*—the family members blame themselves instead of the patient; they feel that everything is their fault and they feel sorry for the person who is ill.

Those who have high expressed emotion tend to be more negative than those whose expressed emotion is low. The attitudes of the relatives determine the direction of the patient's illness after treatment. The relatives influence the outcome of the disorder through negative comments and non-verbal actions. These particular interactions between family members who are dealing with a patient with a psychological disorder are stressful for the recovering patient. The pressure from the family for the patient to recover and to end certain behaviours can cause that person to have a relapse of their illness.

**Further reading**

Piercy FP et al. *Family Therapy Source Book*, 2nd edn. The Guilford Press: New York, 1996.
Rasheed JM and Keung HM. *Family Therapy for Ethnic Minorities*. Sage Publications: London, 2003.

## Systemic approaches

Systemic approaches draw on general systems theory as well as family therapy in order to understand communication within families as well as looking at the wider social context. An individual's behaviour is influenced and maintained by how the family members behave towards each other.

Although systemic approaches were initially developed for working with families, they can also be used with couples.

A genogram or a family tree can provide a useful visual representation of relationships across the generations.

### Concepts that inform practice

*Hypothesizing*

This involves using the information available to generate ideas about how a problem is located in the family. It begins with the information contained in the referral, and continues by using the behaviour of the family during the session.

*Circularity*

This is a questioning technique, used as part of the interview process, to examine the relationship between people. Family members are asked for their view on how other members relate to each other. This reveals repetitive patterns of behaviour and communication between individuals. Asking for each person's view helps to engage all of the participants.

*Neutrality*

The concept of neutrality is a pragmatic one that enables the therapist to hear multiple perspectives without taking sides. It is important to prevent any bias, as it is the system, rather than any one individual, that is the target of change.

### Sessions

Systemic approaches are characterized by team working. Conventionally, this approach uses a one-way screen that separates the therapist and the family from the rest of the team. During a break, the team can feed back their observations and impressions, either to the therapist or directly to the family.

The therapist may give the feedback to the family in the form of 'messages'. These are succinct statements that can be classified as follows:

- *supportive*—for example, commenting positively on communication between the family members
- *hypothesis related*—relaying information about members taking on particular roles for the family
- *prescriptive*—for example, giving the family a specific task.

### Further reading

Dallos R and Draper R. *An Introduction to Family Therapy*. Open University Press: Buckingham, 2000.

# Dialectic behavioural therapy

Dialectic behavioural therapy (DBT) was developed following unsuccessful attempts to apply CBT to a group of young women who all fulfilled the criteria for a diagnosis of borderline personality disorder.

Three sets of strategies and their theories form the three foundations of DBT:

- Validation and acceptance-based strategies help the client to see that their thoughts, feelings, and behaviour are 'normal'. This helps them to realize that they have sound judgement, and to learn how and when to trust themselves.
- Change-based strategies emphasize to clients that change must occur if they are to build a better life for themselves.
- Dialectic strategies allow the therapist to balance acceptance and change in each session, and enable the sessions to move on with speed, movement, and flow. This prevents clients from becoming 'stuck' in rigid thoughts, feelings, and behaviours.

## Functions and modes

Linehan[1] hypothesized that any successful therapy must have five critical functions. It must:

- enhance and maintain the client's motivation to change
- enhance the client's capabilities
- ensure that the client's new capabilities are generalized
- enhance the therapist's motivation to treat clients, while enhancing the therapist's capabilities
- structure the environment so that the treatment can take place.

The individual therapist maintains the client's motivation for treatment. Clients' skills are acquired, developed, strengthened, and generalized through skills training groups, telephone coaching, vivo coaching, and homework assignments. Therapists avoid burnout by having weekly meetings with a consultation team who provide both leadership and support to individual therapists. Therapists and clients meet with families to ensure that adaptive behaviours are being rewarded rather than maladaptive ones being reinforced.

## Stages and targets

To prevent DBT sliding into a treatment that addresses the crisis of the moment week after week, there are specific targets and stages to be followed:

- The first target of the first stage addresses behaviours that could lead to the client's death.
- The second target of the first stage addresses behaviours that lead to the client stopping treatment.
- The third target of the first stage is to build a better quality of life through the acquisition of new skills.

The second stage is to build on all of the targets of the first stage. For example, if the first target was to stop self-harming, the second stage would be to move on from quiet desperation to full emotional experiencing. PTSD would be treated in this stage.

The third stage focuses on the problems of living, the goal being that the client has a normal life of happiness and unhappiness.

The fourth stage has to be designed for clients who do not have a sense of connectedness with a greater whole. The goal is that they develop an ongoing capacity to experience joy and freedom, and that they move away from a sense of incompleteness.

## Reference

1 Linehan M. *Cognitive Behavioural Therapy for Borderline Personality Disorder*. The Guilford Press: New York, 1993.

## Further reading

The Linehan Institute. ℅ www.behavioraltech.org

DeVylder, JE. Dialectical behaviour therapy for the treatment of Borderline Personality Disorder: an evaluation of the evidence. *International Journal of Psychosocial Rehabilitation* 2010:**15**(1): 61–70.

# Gestalt therapy

Gestalt therapy is a form of psychotherapy based on the experiential idea of the 'here and now', and on the relationship that an individual has with others and their environment. The practice of Gestalt therapy is based on personal experience, and an awareness of feelings and behaviour is at its centre. The aim is to help the client to gain greater independence in their actions and overcome any blockages to their development.

## Assumptions

- You cannot work with the mind without taking the body into account—particular emotions are associated with certain postures (e.g. sad, unhappy, withdrawn emotions are associated with reduced eye contact and barriers such as crossed arms).
- An individual is not aware of the entirety of self—they will only be aware of the role they are in at a particular point in time (e.g. patient, professional), to the exclusion of other roles (e.g. mother).
- The mind works on at least two different levels—that which is in the forefront and that which is in the background (e.g. pain in the forefront will take priority over all other activities or obligations until it has resolved).

## How the therapist works

- They expose excessive concentration on past events or future plans, in order to focus on what is in the present (actuality).
- They encourage awareness of thoughts, feelings, body posture, breathing rhythm, and physical sensations, thereby enhancing the client's day-to-day experience (attention).
- They encourage experimentation using dramatization, involving people who are currently significant to the client brought as significant material to the session by the client.
- They replace the concept of blame with the responsibility to create flexibility within relationships.
- They use the five key concepts of awareness:
  - *contact*—individual interpretation of what is going on, as opposed to the perspective of others
  - *sensing*—touching, feeling, auditory, and visual perception (close sensing), thoughts, dreams, body sensations, and emotions (proprioception)
  - *excitement*—a range of emotional and physiological reactions that connect our senses to what is happening in the immediate environment
  - *figure formation*—the way that a central focus of interest emerges
  - *wholeness*—the holistic approach in which the whole is greater than the sum of its parts.

## Key properties of Gestalt therapy

- *Emergence*—becoming visible or apparent; the 'light-bulb' moment.
- *Reification*—treating an abstract concept as if it were real.
- *Multistability*—alternating between two or more mutually exclusive states over time (e.g. role clarification).
- *Invariance*—developing a quality of being that is resistant to variation, an acceptance that 'you are what you are'.

## Further reading

Houston G. *Brief Gestalt Therapy*. Sage Publications: London, 2003.
Polster E and Polster M. *Gestalt Therapy Integrated: contours of theory and practice*. Random House: New York, 1974.

## Psychodynamic therapy

Psychodynamic therapy is a type of psychoanalytic therapy that aims to help people to understand the roots of their emotional distress, often by exploring their unconscious motives, needs, and defences. Put simply, psychodynamic therapy teaches a person to be honest about their feelings. It is one of several mainstream therapies that focus on aspects of the personality, and it is used to treat a variety of conditions, such as depression and personality disorders. Psychodynamic approaches are based on the idea of maladapted functions (moods, behaviours, reactions) developed early in life, which are at least in part unconscious. Therapy sessions have strict boundaries to preserve the sanctity of the therapeutic hour.

### How a psychodynamic therapist works

- The therapist develops a relationship with the client which aims to explore their subconscious mind. In order to do this the therapist must have an in-depth knowledge of him- or herself as a person so as to be aware of any counter-transference (see later in this section).
- The therapist enables the development of trust and understanding in the therapeutic relationship by first addressing the anxiety associated with the maladaptive function.
- The therapist employs free association and free-floating attention involving a great deal of introspection and reflection by the client.
- The therapist reflects how the client is feeling—through words and behaviour—working through resistance and defence mechanisms.
- The therapist uses transference and counter-transference (see later in this section).
- The therapist facilitates insights and understanding by linking the past and the present.
- The therapist interprets the client's communications as images and descriptions.
- The therapist interprets any transference in terms of past relationships.

There are two key dimensions to psychodynamic therapy:

1. *Human development*
- Consideration of the development of individuals from childhood, through adolescence and into adult life, in particular the first 5–6 years (formative years).
- Consideration of past human development in general, and in relation to the personal history of the client. History taking with the client is an essential initial activity.

2. *Personality structure*
- Addressing the basic conflicts that can exist between desires and needs.
- Exploring the internalized sense of what is right and what is wrong.
- Acting as a mediator within the demands of the external world (e.g. role clarification).
- Challenging the two main defence mechanisms—those that deny reality and those that distort reality.

*Transference* refers to the unconscious tendency of a person to assign to others in the present those feelings and attitudes that were originally linked with significant figures in their early life. This might take the form of identifying the therapist with a parent, and may be negative (hostile) or positive (affectionate).

*Counter-transference* occurs when the therapist unconsciously begins to transfer their own repressed feelings on to their client.

## Further reading

Dryden W. *Handbook of Individual Therapies*. Sage Publications: London, 2002.
Jacobs M. *The Presenting Past: the core of psychodynamic counselling and therapy*. Open University Press: Maidenhead, 2006.

# Creative therapies

The creative therapies use artistic interventions and creative processes in therapeutic, rehabilitative, community, and educational settings to promote health, communication, and expression. They aim to foster the integration of physical, emotional, cognitive, and social functioning, to enhance self-awareness, and to facilitate change.

As with all therapies, the relationship between the therapist and the client is of central importance. Creative therapies differ from other psychological therapies in that there is a three-way process between the client, the therapist, and the creative process or intervention. These therapies offer an opportunity for expression and communication with people who find it particularly difficult to express their thoughts and feelings verbally. All creative therapies should be practised by trained and qualified therapists.

Creative therapies can be used with individuals, couples, families, and groups.

## Art therapy

This involves using art materials for self-expression and reflection in the presence of a trained art therapist. Clients who are referred to an art therapist do not need to have previous experience or skill in art, as the therapist is not primarily concerned with making an aesthetic assessment of the image that is created by the client. The overall aim is to enable the client to change and grow on a personal level, by using the affective properties of different art materials in a safe and facilitating environment.

## Music therapy

Music therapists use both instrumental and vocal strategies to facilitate changes that are non-musical in nature. It promotes physical rehabilitation by facilitating movement, increasing motivation to become engaged in treatment, and providing an emotional catharsis and an outlet for expressing feelings. It can also be applied in reminiscence and orientation work with the elderly, through listening and song writing.

## Bibliotherapy

Developmental interactive bibliotherapy refers to the use of literature, discussion, and creative writing in mental illness prevention as well as for assessment, stimulation, and orientation. It promotes understanding, self-expression, self-esteem, and interpersonal skills, and can help people to find new meaning through new ideas, insights, and information. Poetry can be used to promote self-expression, catharsis, and personal growth.

## Drama therapy

Drama therapy is the systematic and intentional use of processes from drama or theatre to achieve the therapeutic goals of symptom relief, emotional and physical integration, and personal growth. It is an active approach that allows the client to tell their story, solve a problem, achieve catharsis, extend the breadth and depth of an inner experience, understand the meaning of images, and strengthen their ability to observe personal roles while increasing flexibility between roles.

## Dance therapy

Dance or movement therapy is the use of movement to further the emotional, cognitive, and physical integration of an individual. It is based on the assumption that the body and the mind are interrelated. It involves direct expression through the body, and is therefore a powerful medium for therapy. Dance therapy can produce changes in feelings, cognition, physical functioning, and behaviour.

## Further reading

Atkinson K and Wells C. *Creative Therapies: a psychodynamic approach within occupational therapy.* Nelson Thornes: Cheltenham, 2000.

Jennings M. *The Map of Your Mind: journeys into creative expression.* McClelland & Stewart Ltd: Plattsburgh, NY, 2001.

## Self-help

Self-help (sometimes called self-management or self-care) is a way of delivering information, interventions and support to people with a range of mental health problems. It is most commonly used to assist people with common mental health problems in primary care, such as anxiety and depression but is also used for people with eating problems, bipolar disorder and other serious mental health problems.

Whilst there is no one agreed definition, professionals tend to value self-help for its emphasis on techniques, manuals and reducing the time they spend delivering traditional psychological therapies. In contrast, mental health service users and patients often define self-help from a recovery orientated philosophy. Here, self-help includes widespread lifestyle strategies, social networks and empowered and informed negotiations with health care professionals.

As an intervention, self-help can be delivered in many formats—leaflets, books, manuals, CD-ROMS, audio or video tapes, interactive automated telephone services and web-based internet programmes. The content and quality of self-help resources is very variable, although the most recent are based on cognitive-behaviour therapy, since this has a good evidence base and is sufficiently structured to make manualisation relatively easy.

### Supporting self-help

Supporting people in using self-help is critical to its effectiveness. Self-help materials may have less benefit without some form of support and guidance, although some computerized self-help programmes mimic a therapist's behaviour and are effective with minimal guidance.

In guided self-help (GSH), nurses should be extremely familiar with the materials that they are supporting. Therapeutic contacts will be brief, and sometimes on the telephone, so nurses should be highly skilled in developing a rapid therapeutic alliance, initially engaging the person and then developing and maintaining that alliance, despite the brevity of contact. It is more effective to have short but frequent contacts than to have a few long contacts.

Self-help should be situated within a 'stepped care' system. Although it may be useful for some people, others who are not improving will need to be 'stepped up' to traditional psychological therapy or psychiatric care. Decisions about stepping up should be the result of a scheduled review, supported by standardized outcome measures, where the nurse and the client can discuss the next stage of a shared plan.

### Further reading

Lovell K, Richards DA and Bower P. Improving access to primary mental health care: uncontrolled evaluation of a pilot self-help clinic. *British Journal of General Practice* 2003; 53: 133–5.

National Institute for Health and Care Excellence (NICE). *Depression: management of depression in primary and secondary care.* CG23. NICE: London, 2004.

## Complementary therapies

These are therapies that are not part of orthodox medical treatment. They are not usually administered by a medically trained practitioner, and are not normally available in a traditional hospital setting (although some, such as acupuncture, are available in NHS hospitals, where they are administered by qualified practitioners who may or may not be medically trained). Complementary therapies can be used alongside or instead of traditional medicine. However, some of these treatments can interact with traditional medicine, and this can sometimes cause complications. A complementary therapy should only be administered by a practitioner who is fully trained in that particular therapy, and following a comprehensive health assessment.

Complementary therapies have been used for many centuries, and some of these treatments are the foundations of the traditional medicines that we use today.

### Herbalism

Herbs have been used as medicines since the dawn of human history, and many common drugs are made from herbal extracts. The natural chemical properties of certain herbs have been shown to be of medicinal value. However, in contrast to conventional medicine, herbalists use the 'whole' herb or plant, rather than isolating and breaking down chemical compounds and then synthesizing other compounds from them. This is because the plant, being a part of nature, is said to represent perfect balance—therefore healing requires the natural combination of elements in the plant or herb, not just a single chemical within it.

### Homeopathy

Homeopathy was developed in the eighteenth century by Samuel Hahemann (1753–1843). It is based on the belief that 'like cures like'. Remedies are derived from plants, animals, and minerals. These are diluted and then administered in minute doses. The idea is that the same substance that causes symptoms if given to a healthy person can be used in much smaller doses to cure someone who is unwell. For example, caffeine given to a healthy person causes central nervous system stimulation and increased urine output. Caffeine given in much smaller doses could be used in homeopathy for someone who complains of excess urine output, sleeplessness, and unusual mental activity.

Homeopathy strives to treat the cause of the illness, not the symptoms, thus preventing a recurrence of illness.

### Reiki

Reiki was developed in Japan by Mikao Usui, and was brought to the West in the 1930s. It is a gentle non-invasive technique, based on channelling energy through seven major chakras or energy centres in the body to treat physical and emotional ailments. The practitioner does not touch their client, but moves their hands a few centimetres above the body, slowly moving over the entire body in order to detect the areas of heat, which are the areas that need treatment. Opening up the chakras allows the energy meridians to flow and balances the body's energy, restoring a healthy aura, and thus a healthy body.

## Reflexology

This is the technique of applying gentle pressure to reflexes in both hands and feet. These reflexes correspond to particular parts of the body. When stimulated, these parts of the nervous system cause responses in the relevant parts of the body to promote a feeling of deep relaxation, and the subsequent restoration of balance in the body brings healing. Balance can be lost through prolonged stress and illness.

## Acupuncture

Acupuncture is based on beliefs in Chinese and Eastern medicine about a motivating energy source called 'Qi'. This energy source needs to be able to move through the body in a balanced, smooth way through a series of meridians or chakras under the skin. When the flow of energy is unbalanced, illness ensues. By inserting fine needles into the channels of energy, the acupuncturist can stimulate the body's own healing process. This achieves physical, emotional, and spiritual balance in the individual.

## Shiatsu

This is a Japanese technique of massage, based on similar principles of using the energy flow or meridians in the body. The shiatsu practitioner uses a series of gentle holding techniques, pressing with the palms, thumbs, elbows, knees, and feet on the meridians. When appropriate, more dynamic rotations and stretches are used. Once energy flow has been restored, good health is the result.

## Further reading

Springhouse. *Nurse's Handbook of Alternative and Complementary Therapies*, 2nd edn. Lippincott Williams & Wilkins: Philadelphia, PA, 2002.

# Psychosocial interventions for psychoses

Over the last 50 years considerable research has been done both to improve our understanding of psychosis, and to identify effective interventions to support the recovery of those who experience psychosis. As a result of this research, outcomes for this patient group have significantly improved, and psychosis and schizophrenia are now treated optimistically with psychosocial interventions.[2] These have been defined as follows:[3,4]

- using a collaborative partnership with the recovery paradigm at the core
- interventions that span and integrate a range of medical, social, and psychological evidence-based interventions
- interventions that include at least one of the evidence-based components that are described below.

## An integrated biopsychosocial model of psychosis[5] (taught within a stress-vulnerability model of psychosis)

### Cognitive behavioural approaches

CBT is a psychological intervention that was originally developed for the treatment of depression. It is based on the premise that our thoughts affect our feelings and subsequent behaviour. CBT has been adapted and extensively used in the management of schizophrenia and related psychoses, with impressive outcomes. The main aim of CBT is to address the distress that psychotic symptoms cause to the affected individual, rather than to reduce the symptoms per se. CBT aims to help the individual to normalize and make sense of their psychotic experiences as a way of improving their functioning and quality of life.

### Psychological management of symptoms

Emphasis is placed on establishing a therapeutic alliance between the mental health professional and the person with psychosis, which facilitates understanding of the person and their difficulties, provides support during challenges (e.g. relapse), and promotes stability and adaptation. Some of the therapeutic techniques that are used include emphatic validation, praise, advice, very gentle confrontation, psychoeducation (including identifying and managing early signs of relapse), promoting self-awareness and self-management, and fostering personal growth.

### Cognitive behavioural family interventions

These interventions were developed from studies that explored why people returning to some environments relapsed more frequently than others (within the first 9 months following discharge). The term 'expressed emotion (EE)' was coined, with high EE describing the situation in which people were exposed to criticism, over-involvement, and hostility, and low EE where there was warmth and more positive coping strategies. These findings led to the development of family intervention to increase social functioning, reduce the care burden on families, improve the quality of life of people with psychosis, and reduce the rate of relapse. The intervention includes engaging families, assessing need, improving communication, and problem solving.[6]

The success of family intervention studies has provided support for the emerging understanding that people with psychosis do not recover without supportive environments, and it has also promoted support and skills development in family groups,[7] and highlighted sibling needs.[8]

*Medication management*

See Chapter 2.

With regard to the treatment and management of psychosis and schizophrenia,[9] the National Institute for Health and Care Excellence (NICE) recommends that mental health services should promote carer inclusion, peer support and self-management, and recovery by routinely offering:

- crisis and risk management
- assessment (including PTSD) and engagement
- psychological and pharmacological intervention
- physical health monitoring and guidance.

## Benefits of using psychosocial interventions[10–12]

*For clients*

- Improved biopsychosocial outcomes.
- Improved collaboration, involvement, and empowerment.

*For carers*

- Improved knowledge and awareness.
- Reduction in 'EE' and care burden.
- Increased satisfaction with services.

*For professionals*

- Promotion and/or new opportunities.
- Acquisition of knowledge and skills.
- Positive attitudes to and beliefs about psychosis.

## References

2 National Institute for Health and Care Excellence (NICE). *Psychosis and Schizophrenia in Adults: treatment and management.* CG178. NICE: London, 2014. ✍ www.nice.org.uk/CG178

3 Sin J and Scully E. An evaluation of education and implementation of psychosocial interventions within one UK mental healthcare trust. *Journal of Psychiatric and Mental Health Nursing* 2008; **15**: 161–9.

4 Brooker C and Brabban A. *Measured Success: a scoping review of evaluated psychosocial interventions training for work with people with serious mental health problems.* National Institute for Mental Health in England: Mansfield, 2004.

5 Gamble C and Brennan G. *Working with Serious Mental Illness: a manual for clinical practice,* 2nd edn. Elsevier: London, 2006.

6 Askey R, Gamble C and Gray R. Family work in first-onset psychosis: a literature review. *Journal of Psychiatric and Mental Health Nursing* 2007; **14**: 356–65.

7 Gamble C and Sin J. Developing whole systems recovery programmes for families. *Early Intervention in Psychiatry* 2014; **8 (Suppl. 1)**: 1–168.

8 Sin J et al. Making connections with families: how inclusive are England's EIPS? *Early Intervention in Psychiatry* 2014; **8 (Suppl. 1)**: 1–168.

9 National Institute for Health and Care Excellence (NICE). *Psychosis and Schizophrenia in Adults: treatment and management.* CG178. NICE: London, 2014. ✍ www.nice.org.uk/CG178

10 Sin J and Scully E. An evaluation of education and implementation of psychosocial interventions within one UK mental healthcare trust. *Journal of Psychiatric and Mental Health Nursing* 2008; **15**: 161–9.

11 Gamble C and Brennan G. *Working with Serious Mental Illness: a manual for clinical practice,* 2nd edn. Elsevier: London, 2006.

12 Brooker C and Brabban A. *Measured Success: a scoping review of evaluated psychosocial interventions training for work with people with serious mental health problems.* National Institute for Mental Health in England: Mansfield, 2004.

## Further reading

Bentall R. *Madness Explained: psychosis and human nature.* Penguin: London, 2004. (Richard Bentall normalizes the dividing line between mental health and mental illness. He maintains that severe mental disorders can no longer be reduced to brain chemistry, but must be understood psychologically, as part of normal behaviour and human nature—hence the value of routinely using psychosocial interventions.)

Lobban F and Barrowclough C. *A Casebook of Family Interventions for Psychosis.* John Wiley & Sons Ltd: Chichester, 2009. (This guide to family interventions illustrates different family intervention approaches. It outlines how to tailor them to meet different needs—for example, working via an interpreter, or with families in which multiple members have mental health problems.)

## Useful websites

Meriden Family Programme: ✍ www.meridenfamilyprogramme.com
(This site provides useful information and resources for carers, family members, friends, mental health professionals, and commissioners.)

Rethink Mental Illness: ✍ www.rethink.org/home
(This site helps people who are living with psychosis and schizophrenia. It also provides an excellent resource to support siblings and introduce them to the Siblings Network at ✍ www.rethink.org/carers-family-friends/brothers-and-sisters-siblings-network)

# Behavioural activation

Behavioural activation (BA) is a structured psychological treatment for depression. Its theoretical basis is that depression is best understood as a functional problem, and that altering the external context rather than internal factors (such as a person's thoughts) is likely to lead to improvement.

According to behavioural theory, the behaviours associated with depression lead to a reduction in opportunities for people to experience pleasure (positive reinforcement), while rewarding avoidance (negative reinforcement). When depression strikes, people withdraw from situations and activities that give them negative feelings, and they find it increasingly hard to return to these activities. This reduces the possibility that they will have pleasant experiences. Depressive behaviours make depression worse.

## Treatment

Although BA is often used in CBT as the first stage of treatment, research trials have shown that when BA is used as a stand-alone treatment it is just as effective as CBT, cognitive therapy, or antidepressants. BA is also the essential component of problem-solving treatment for depression, and has been used successfully in many collaborative care and self-help trials.

Essentially, BA targets avoidance behaviour. It identifies the activities which a depressed person has reduced in their life. These can be categorized into routine, pleasurable, and necessary activities. Routine activities are those (often mundane) things we do that 'anchor' our lives—activities such as shopping, cleaning, cooking, and getting up at the same time every day. Pleasurable activities include private leisure (e.g. reading the newspaper) and social pursuits (e.g. talking to friends). Necessary activities (e.g. dealing with a conflict at work, paying bills, filling in forms) are often aversive.

People start BA by compiling three separate lists of routine, pleasurable, and necessary activities. They then make a hierarchical list consisting of a mixture of all three types of activities, from easiest to hardest. Finally, activities are selected from low down the list and weekly plans are developed to reactivate them. Each week the diaries are reviewed and new activities are scheduled.

## Supporting behavioural activation

Nurses and other mental health professionals can support patients using BA. It is easy to teach, and highly acceptable to patients and workers. Telephone support can often be effective, so long as some face-to-face education sessions and good-quality information manuals have been provided previously. Recently studies have shown that nurses are highly effective in supporting and treating people depression using BA.

## Further reading

Ekers D, Webster L, Van Straten A, Cuijpers P, Richards D, et al. Behavioural Activation for Depression; An update of Meta-Analysis of Effectiveness and Sub-group Analysis. *PLos ONE* 2014; 9(6): e100100.

Ekers D, Richarols DA, McMillan D, Bland JM and Gilbody S. Behavioural activation delivered by the non-specialist: phase II randomized controlled trial. *British Journal of Psychiatry* 2011; 198: 66–72.

Jacobson NS, Martell CR and Dimidjian S. Behavioral activation treatment for depression: returning to contextual roots. *Clinical Psychology: Science and Practice* 2001; 8: 255–70.

Richards D. Behavioural activation. In: J Bennett-Levy et al. (eds) *Oxford Guide to Low Intensity CBT Interventions*. Oxford University Press: Oxford, 2010. pp. 141–50.

# Relapse prevention

Relapse prevention in mental health can be divided into three areas—pharmacological, psychological, and combination approaches. Combination approaches are the preferred option.

## Pharmacological relapse prevention

At least 45% of people who are diagnosed with schizophrenia or bipolar affective disorder do not take their medication as prescribed. This problem is not unique to individuals with mental health problems—similar levels of non-compliance with medication are found in the treatment of tuberculosis, diabetes, and leprosy.

Non-compliance with medication is thought to increase the risk of relapse in schizophrenia by at least fourfold. In bipolar disorder, non-compliance with medication is the most robust predictor of subsequent hospital admission, considerably above all other causative factors.

Pharmacological relapse prevention shares many of the fundamental precepts of medication management (see Chapter 2). Any medication prescription regimen that aims to prevent relapse due to medication non-compliance should be decided jointly by the prescriber, the service user, and any mental health practitioner who is in close regular contact with the service user. This will reduce non-compliance due to matters such as medication side effects, health beliefs, and cultural preferences.

Factors that are relevant to pharmacological relapse prevention include:
- the joint planning of a medication regimen
- the suitability of the prescribed medication profile
- analysis of barriers to adherence and problem solving
- motivational interviewing to eradicate or reduce these barriers.

## Psychological relapse prevention

Research consistently shows that even when service users are fully compliant with medication, breakthrough episodes of illness are the norm. Medication alone is thought to prevent relapse in only 30–50% of individuals with a psychotic disorder, and the figures are similar for those with mood disorders.

It is therefore clear that relapse prevention based solely on promoting adherence to medication is insufficient for at least 50% of all service users, and that psychological strategies aimed at minimizing relapse are equally important.

There are a number of models of psychological relapse prevention, and central to each of them is the concept of prodrome management. The word 'prodrome' is derived from the Greek word 'prodromos', which means the forerunner of an event.

### Prodrome management or early warning signs management

Service users are encouraged to identify individual early signs that an illness episode may be imminent. These signs may be physical (sleeplessness), behavioural (a change in behavioural routine), affective (emergence of mood associated with an illness episode), or cognitive (alteration in cognitive mechanisms, such as appraisal of danger). Prodromes vary between individuals, but tend to be consistent for each individual.

*Prodrome recognition therapy*

Service users are asked to identify their own early warning signs, often from a list or card sort.[13] This list is then refined, often with the help of family, friends, or mental health workers. Early signs are then ranked according to the point at which they occur in an episode—at the beginning, middle, or end. Once the prodrome list has been established, an action plan is devised that details what action should be taken when a prodrome is identified, to prevent the onset of a full episode of illness.

Each action plan is tailored to the needs of the individual service user, and may include factors such as behavioural change, change to medication, or the promotion of awareness of cognitive biases or misinterpretations. The promotion of assistance seeking on identification of a prodrome is particularly important.

## Combined approaches

Combined approaches are simply a combination of pharmacological and psychological relapse prevention plans, and are in most cases the preferred option.

## Reference

13 Perry A et al. Randomized controlled trial of the efficacy of teaching patients with bipolar disorder to identify early symptoms of relapse and obtain treatment. *British Medical Journal* 1999; **318**: 139–53.

## Further reading

Kennard BD et al. Sequential treatment with fluoxetine and relapse-prevention CBT to improve outcomes in pediatric depression. *American Journal of Psychiatry* 2014; **171**: 1083–90.

Witkiewitz K and Marlatt GA. Relapse prevention for alcohol and drug problems: that was Zen, this is Tao. *American Psychologist* 2004; **59**: 224–35.

# Assertive outreach teams

### Client group

Assertive outreach teams (AOTs) aim to meet the needs of people with high levels of disability associated with severe and persistent mental health problems such as schizophrenia. Users of assertive outreach services typically have a history of frequent inpatient admissions and complex multiple needs, including the risk of self-harm, persistent offending, substance misuse, or insecure accommodation. Most assertive outreach service users have a history of difficulties in maintaining lasting and consenting contact with services.

### Team purpose

These teams initially focus on engagement, by providing ongoing support to the client, their carer, or their family. As therapeutic alliances develop, they aim to reduce hospital admissions, lengths of stay, and symptom severity, and to improve social functioning.

Assertive outreach is not an intervention in itself, but it is a platform from which interventions are delivered. A future challenge for AOTs is the integration of vocational, employment, and other socially rehabilitative interventions into existing service provision.

The term 'assertive' implies a tenacious and persistent approach rather than an aggressive one, emphasizing the need for creative interventions that foster engagement.

### Team characteristics and principles

AOTs differ in terms of size, staff composition, and the service sector in which they are based. They originate from within mainstream psychiatry, but an increasing number of AOTs now operate from the voluntary sector. Differences between statutory and voluntary sector services are often unclear. Voluntary sector services tend not to hold formal clinical responsibility, and are smaller, contain fewer staff disciplines, and have no control over inpatient bed usage.

Recommended principles of assertive outreach care include the following:
* a self-contained service that is responsible for a wide range of interventions
* a single responsible medical officer as an active team member
* a long-term treatment emphasizing continuity of care
* most services delivered in community settings
* ongoing contact and relationship building with service users
* overall care coordination responsibility
* small caseloads of no more than 12 clients per worker.

## Outcomes

- Increased engagement.
- Improved service user satisfaction.
- No differences in admission rates, clinical or social outcomes.
- Little differences in costs compared to other approaches.

## Further reading

Burns T and Firn M. *Assertive Outreach in Mental Health: a manual for practitioners.* Oxford University Press: Oxford, 2002.

# Early intervention in psychosis

An early recognition of psychosis allows early intervention and the initiation of appropriate treatment and management strategies. Delays can have serious consequences for both the patient and their family.

## Benefits of early intervention

Studies of early intervention demonstrate that it reduces the risk of people developing a florid psychosis. In addition, with early intervention they may experience:

- more rapid recovery
- a better prognosis
- preservation of psychosocial skills
- preservation of family and social support
- maintenance of social and educational status
- reduced need for hospitalization
- more effective treatment within the 'critical period' (see 'Risks' section on p. 135)
- reduced duration of untreated illness.

## Epidemiology of psychosis

The risk factors for psychotic illness include old age, adolescence, and young adulthood. They also include existing traits and vulnerabilities, such as:

- family history of mental illness
- vulnerable personality (e.g. schizoid personality type)
- delayed milestones (walking, talking)
- low intelligence
- history of obstetric or perinatal complications
- winter birth
- stress factors, including life events, perceived psychosocial stress, substance misuse, and subjective or functional changes.

## History of early intervention in psychosis

Delays in treatment result in significant distress for patients, as well as incomplete recovery, poorer prognosis, higher suicide risk, substance misuse, and enduring levels of social disability. Delays in receiving treatment are independently associated with a greatly increased risk of relapse.

The 'prodrome' has been identified as a period of non-psychotic disturbance that occurs just before the emergence of a psychotic episode. If the patient is left undiagnosed and untreated they will go on to develop a psychotic illness. However, if the prodrome can be recognized, and treatment offered, it may be possible to halt the progression to a psychotic illness. Delays in treatment of up to a year have been reported, often characterized by unavailable care pathways and signs going unrecognized.

## Clinical features of the prodrome or pre-psychotic state

Adolescents and young adults are in a highly transitory life stage. However, the persistent presence of the following signs over a 2-week period should arouse suspicion that the patient may be in an 'at-risk' mental state:

- suspiciousness
- depression
- anxiety and tension
- irritability
- anger
- mood swings
- sleep disturbances
- appetite changes
- loss of energy or motivation
- the perception that things around them have altered
- the belief that things have speeded up or slowed down
- deterioration in work or educational performance
- lack of interest in socializing
- emergence of unusual beliefs (e.g. magical thinking).

These signs may be present in stress and other disorders. An unexplained loss of social function or a sustained lack of contact with peers should arouse further suspicion.

## Principles of early intervention

These include:

- treatment of psychotic symptoms with low-dose atypical antipsychotic medication
- treatment of accompanying anxiety or depression
- gaining the patient's trust, to promote compliance with antipsychotic treatment (psychoeducation)
- making an effort to minimize distress associated with hospitalization and treatment
- involving the patient's family and friends in the recovery plan, being mindful of the phasic nature of the illness, and using a staged approach.

## Risks

One in five young men with adolescent-onset schizophrenia commits suicide. Around 70% of young suicides involve substance misuse. The critical period from the onset of psychoses to schizophrenia is 2–5 years. An inadequate and untimely treatment period increases the duration of untreated psychoses. This leads to increased risk of relapse, residual symptoms, social disability, and reduced quality of life.

## Outcomes

- Improved prodromal symptoms.
- Improved employment and family therapy gains.
- Quality of evidence variable.

## Further reading

Edwards J and McGorry P. *Implementing Early Intervention in Psychosis: a guide to establishing early psychosis services.* Martin Dunitz Ltd: London, 2002.

Marshall M and Rathbone J. Early intervention for psychosis. *Cochrane Database of Systematic Reviews* 2011; 6:CD004718.

# Group therapy

Group therapy is an intervention in which ideally around 8 to 10 people meet together to discuss issues that are causing them concern.

## The aims of group therapy

Group therapy gives members an opportunity to:

- try out new ways of behaving
- learn more about the way that they interact with others
- share their feelings and thoughts in an open and honest manner
- develop trust in working with others
- learn how to work with others
- receive feedback from others on how they relate to others
- interact freely with others
- resolve the issues that led to them seeking help
- provide support to and receive support from others
- help themselves and others to find healthy alternatives to troubling issues
- develop new skills in relating to people.

## Indications for group therapy

Group therapy is indicated for people who:

- wish to explore issues in a context that is closer to real life
- welcome the opportunity to reflect on their own and others' interpersonal skills
- will benefit from active participation with others
- want feedback from others on issues that are troubling them
- have deficits in their interpersonal and social skills
- have problems developing trust in working with others
- want to learn more about how they interact with others
- want to learn more about how they relate to others.

## The effectiveness of group therapy

There is evidence from well-designed studies that group therapy leads to successful outcomes for people living with mental health problems, including depression, anorexia nervosa, schizophrenia, and alcohol dependency, and for suicidal adolescents.

## Further reading

Roth A and Fonagy P. *What Works for Whom? A critical review of psychotherapy research*, 2nd edn. The Guilford Press: New York, 2004.
Rutgers College Counselling Centre. *Group Therapy Virtual Brochure*. Available at ✄ www.rci.rutgers.edu

# Joint crisis plans for people with psychosis

Joint crisis plans (JCPs) are a collaborative means of working that is developed between mental health teams and service users. The aim is for the service user and the clinical team to reach agreement through negotiation and consensus building.

Each completed crisis card or plan contains information that includes an assessment of previous crises, as well as an advance plan for care in a crisis. JCPs have psychological value for the carrier/holder, and they are a potential advocacy tool for use during a crisis.

A JCP agreement is achieved prior to any episode of illness, and at a time when the service user is well enough to develop a crisis plan. JCPs (carried by the service user) are thought to be especially useful during a crisis when the individual may be too unwell to articulate any treatment preferences.

This approach has been likened to the advance directives and living wills described in the literature on physical illness.[14]

There is a high rate of relapse among people suffering from psychosis. This may result in numerous admissions to inpatient psychiatric units, and it is distressing for the individuals concerned. JCPs aim to mitigate some of the negative consequences of relapse, including admission to hospital, the use of coercion in the form of the application of the Mental Health Act, and the costs associated with these consequences.

Henderson and colleagues showed that JCPs were able to significantly reduce compulsory inpatient treatment, compared with treatment as usual.[15] JCP users experienced fewer admissions and significantly reduced application of the Mental Health Act. Around 13% of JCP users experienced compulsory admission or treatment, compared with 27% of the control group.

However, the UK's largest trial of JCPs[16] showed that they did not reduce compulsory treatment in people with severe mental illness.

➜ Relapse prevention, p. 130.

## References

14 Stewart K and Bowker L. Advance directives and living wills. *Postgraduate Medical Journal* 1998; **74**: 151–6.
15 Henderson C et al. Effect of joint crisis plans on use of compulsory treatment in psychiatry: single blind randomised controlled trial. *British Medical Journal* 2004; **329**: 136.
16 Thornicroft G et al. Clinical outcomes of Joint Crisis Plans to reduce compulsory treatment for people with psychosis: a randomised controlled trial. *The Lancet* 2013; **381**: 1634–41.

## Further reading

🔊 www.mentalhealthcare.org.uk/media/downloads/CRIMSON_jointcrisisplans.pdf

# Six-category intervention analysis

Six-category intervention analysis is a communication and counselling framework developed by John Heron. It is a tool that enables nurses to select, monitor, and reflect on their communication skills and interactions with their clients. It provides a way of classifying a huge range of skills under six types of interventions which include six kinds of purpose or intention. These intentions underlie the ultimate choice of intervention, and can be applied equally to one-to-one and group communication.

## Interventions

There are three categories of authoritative interventions and three categories of facilitative interventions.

### Authoritative interventions

These are so called because in each case the practitioner is taking a more overtly dominant or assertive role. They place more emphasis on what the practitioner is doing, and include the following categories:

- *1. Prescriptive*—aiming to direct the behaviour of the client (e.g. to give advice: 'I think you will feel better if you talk about why you are anxious').
- *2. Informative*—aiming to impart new knowledge and information to the client (e.g. to give information: 'These tablets can cause you to feel drowsy').
- *3. Confronting*—aiming to directly challenge the restrictive attitude, belief, or behaviour of the client (e.g. to challenge or give direct feedback: 'Are you aware that when you shout you frighten your family?').

### Facilitative interventions

Facilitative interventions are less obtrusive and more discreet, and the emphasis is on the effect of the intervention on the client. They include the following categories:

- *4. Cathartic*—aiming to enable the client to abreact painful emotion (e.g. to help to release tension or encourage laughter or crying: 'From what you have experienced—I can imagine how angry you may feel').
- *5. Catalytic*—aiming to enable the client to learn and develop by self-direction and self-discovery within the practitioner–client context, but also beyond it (e.g. to encourage self-directed problem solving: 'How do you think you could improve your situation?').
- *6. Supportive*—aiming to affirm the worth and value of the client (e.g. to be approving or validating: 'You really tried to control your anger').

Each of these six categories is value neutral—that is, no one category is more or less important than the others when used in an appropriate context. However, they are only of real value if they are rooted in care and concern for the client.

## Applying six-category intervention analysis

In practice, the skill required of the nurse is to be:
- equally proficient in each of the six categories
- aware of which category they are using and why, at any given time
- able to move skilfully from one type of intervention to any other as required by the developing situation and the purpose of the interaction.

## Further reading

Ashmore R and Banks D. Student nurses' use of their interpersonal skills within clinical role-plays. *Nurse Education Today* 2004; **24**: 20–9.

Heron J. *Helping the Client: a creative practical guide*, 5th edn. Sage Publications: London, 2001.

Morrissey J and Callaghan P. Heron's communication framework: six category intervention analysis. *Communication Skills for Mental Health Nurses*. Open University Press: Maidenhead, 2011. pp. 61–75.

Sloan G and Watson H. John Heron's six-category intervention analysis: towards understanding interpersonal relations and progressing the delivery of clinical supervision for mental health nursing in the United Kingdom. *Journal of Advanced Nursing* 2001; **36**: 206–14.

# An intervention to reduce absconding from acute psychiatric wards

Patients who abscond from acute psychiatric wards evoke anxiety in staff, relatives, and carers. Returning the patient to hospital also takes up valuable staff and police time. Those close to the patient may lose faith in psychiatric services, and, importantly, the patient may deteriorate as a result of loss of contact with psychiatric services.

## An intervention package

Research on absconding by Bowers and colleagues in 1999 provided a basis for the formulation of an intervention package that staff could use to reduce absconding by patients from their wards.[17]

The intervention was tested in a 'before and after' trial in five acute psychiatric wards in 2003. Absconding rates fell by 25% overall during the intervention period. The researchers trained the ward staff in the intervention, which can be summarized as follows.

*Elements of the intervention*
- The use of a signing in and out book so that staff know the location of service users.
- Identification of service users at high risk of absconding.
- Purposeful nursing time with the identified high-risk group.
- Breaking bad news carefully to these patients.
- Debriefing following ward incidents.
- A multidisciplinary review following two absconding events.

Before the project began, the previous research findings and the intervention were explained to the staff by the researchers. The benefits of participation for them and for their patients were explained. This dialogue enabled joint working to identify ways in which the intervention could be implemented. The staff also agreed to collect outcome data.

*Outcome data*
- Data on the frequency of door locking were collected.
- Data on ward incidents were collected with the aid of the Staff Observation Aggression Scale (SOAS).[18]
- Data on the time when absconding occurred were collected.

The intervention commenced on two wards. The staff required considerable support and encouragement with regard to both data collection and implementation of the package. After a cooling-off period the other three wards were supported in implementing the package. At the end of the research project, staff were invited to discuss their experiences during participation in focus groups.

Three wards implemented the intervention successfully, and absconding decreased in two of these wards. For various reasons associated with ward stability, the other two wards did not implement the intervention consistently. Staff on all of the wards became much more aware of the antecedents to absconding events. Anecdotally, several staff members perceived that the ward nursing regimens had become less custodial and more therapeutic as a result of the intervention.

## References

17 Bowers L et al. Absconding: why patients leave. *Journal of Psychiatric and Mental Health Nursing* 1999; 6: 199–205.
18 Nijman H et al. The Staff Observation Aggression Scale–Revised (SOAS-R). *Aggressive Behavior* 1999; 25: 197–203.

## Further reading

Bowers L, Alexander J and Gaskell K. A trial of an anti-absconding intervention in acute psychiatric wards. *Journal of Psychiatric and Mental Health Nursing* 2003; 10: 410–16.

# Electroconvulsive therapy

Electroconvulsive therapy (ECT) is a procedure that involves a brief application of an electric current to the brain, through the scalp, inducing a seizure. It is typically used to treat a person who is experiencing severe depression or acute mania.

ECT remains the most controversial treatment for psychiatric illness, although it has been used since the 1940s and 1950s. Many of the risks and side effects have been related to the misuse of equipment, incorrect administration, and inadequately trained staff. There is also a misconception that ECT is used as a 'quick fix' instead of long-term therapy or hospitalization. Unfavourable news reports and media coverage have added to the controversy surrounding this treatment. ECT is generally safe and is one of the most effective treatments available for intractable depression.

## How ECT is administered

The procedure is performed by an anaesthetist, a psychiatrist, and a qualified ECT nurse.

### Before ECT

General anaesthesia is used for this procedure, so the patient will be advised not to eat or drink before ECT. They will also be given a muscle relaxant, so that there will be no movement of the body during the procedure.

### During ECT

Electrodes are placed on the patient's scalp and a finely controlled electric current is applied, which causes a brief seizure in the brain. Because the muscles are relaxed, the seizure will usually be limited to slight movement of the hands and feet. The patient is carefully monitored during ECT treatment. When they wake up, minutes later, they do not remember the treatment or the events surrounding it, and they may be confused.

### After ECT

Side effects may be caused by the anaesthesia or by the ECT itself, or by both. Immediate side effects that may occur within the first few hours after a treatment include:
• headaches
• muscle aches or muscle soreness
• nausea
• confusion
• hypotension—low blood pressure
• tachycardia—a heart rate that is faster than normal, which may accompany a bounding pulse
• allergic reaction to the anaesthesia
• loss of memory for some events that occurred around the time of the treatment is common. This memory loss improves, but some patients have persistent gaps in memory for that time period. These will need to be monitored by the nurse.

**Further reading**

National Institute for Health and Care Excellence (NICE). *Guidance on the Use of Electro-Convulsive Therapy*. TA59. NICE: London, 2003.

# Challenging behaviour

Challenging behaviour is a term used to describe behavioural distress. It is most often used by those caring for people with learning disabilities, or children and adolescents, but it is also used by those caring for people with mental health problems.

## Definitions

Challenging behaviour is defined as:

> behaviour of such intensity, frequency or duration that the physical safety of the person or others is likely to be placed in serious jeopardy, or behaviour which is likely to seriously limit or deny access to, and use of, ordinary community facilities.[19]

The Mental Health Foundation has expanded on this to include behaviour that is likely to:

> impair an individual's personal development and family life and which represents a challenge to services, to families, and to the individual themselves, however caused.[20]

Within mental health services, challenging behaviour is manifested by the following:

- aggression
- self-injury
- disruption and/or destruction of the environment
- stereotyped or idiosyncratic behaviour.

Examples of these behaviours in people with mental health problems range from intimidating others to self-harming behaviours such as cutting, and regressed behaviours such as refusing to self-care. Mental health professionals may label such behaviours as 'attention-seeking'—this is often an indication of staff frustration and possible power struggles.

## Management of challenging behaviour

Management of challenging behaviour requires an understanding of the underlying motivation. This can be divided into two broad categories—an inability to communicate frustration or a need in a more acceptable manner, or a means of controlling their environment. Any strategy that is designed to manage challenging behaviour must consider that it may be reinforced by the response of others. Strategies for managing challenging behaviour involve setting limits non-punitively. Before setting these limits:

- Ask the carers to state their expectations of the client in a positive way rather than a negative one.
- Explore the reasons for, and meaning of, the behaviour with the client, and consider alternative behaviours.
- Inform the client which behaviours are acceptable and which are not, and explain the consequences of behaving unacceptably.

Once these issues have been clarified with the client, the consequences of unacceptable behaviour must be enforced. Firm, but not hostile, enforcement of limits is essential. Success requires that every member of the care team is consistent in their understanding of, and response to, the limits set. The care team does not assume responsibility for the client's behaviour, whether positive or negative. The client retains the right to choose how he or she behaves, so long as the consequences are clear.

## References

19 Emerson E and Einfeld SL. *Challenging Behaviour*, 3rd edn. Cambridge University Press: Cambridge, 2011.
20 Mental Health Foundation. *Updates* 3: issue 19, June 2002. Available at ℘ www.mentalhealth.org.uk

## Further reading

Emerson E and Einfeld SL. *Challenging Behaviour*. 3rd edn. Cambridge University Press: Cambridge, 2011.

# Assessment of children and adolescents

## Introduction

In order to assess children and adolescents with mental health problems, nurses need to have a good knowledge of child and adolescent development, mental health problems, risk factors, safeguarding procedures, and legal and ethical issues.

The assessment process involves systematically gathering information by asking questions and making observations of the child or adolescent. Information should also be sought from other sources, such as parents and teachers. Together this information enables the nurse to make sense of the presenting problem.

## Assessment frameworks and tools

The Common Assessment Framework[21] offers an integrated approach to assessment and intervention. The Care Programme Approach[22] provides a framework for systematic assessment, formulation and care planning, identifying a key worker, and regular reviews. These generic assessment frameworks can be supplemented with specialist assessments depending on the presenting problem—for example, the Autism Diagnostic Observation Schedule (ADOS), or the Eating Disorders Inventory–3 (EDI-3).

## Nursing skills and values

Core nursing skills and values are needed to conduct an assessment. These include appropriate verbal and non-verbal communication, active listening, being non-judgemental, caring, and forming therapeutic relationships.

## Assessment process

- Prepare a safe space or environment that is conducive to the therapeutic process.
- Ensure access to all the necessary equipment (e.g. assessment forms, leaflets, diary).
- Meet with the child or adolescent on their own.
- Meet with the parent(s) and assess family life and interactions.
- Explain and discuss the parameters of confidentiality.
- Liaison—obtain information from different perspectives from others who know the young person (this should usually be done with the young person's consent).
- Follow a structured assessment format that includes duration, frequency, and intensity of the presenting problem, mental health, physical health, developmental history, family relationships, social life, strengths and resources, and the young person's hopes and aims.
- Take a holistic view of the social, cultural, and environmental context of the child or adolescent.
- Work collaboratively with the young person and their parents.
- Combine your knowledge and the evidence base with your understanding of the individual.
- Follow principles of good record keeping and clear documentation.
- Discuss the assessment with colleagues as part of the consultation process and in clinical supervision.

## Formulation

A formulation organizes the information obtained from the assessment and provides an explanation, undertaken in consultation and collaboration with the child or adolescent and their parents. It gives meaning to the issues explored in the assessment process and informs the intervention.

One formulation framework used in CBT and other models is that of the 'five Ps'—presenting issues, precipitating factors, perpetuating factors, predisposing factors, and protective factors (see Table 4.1).

**Table 4.1** The five Ps: formulation

| Presenting issues | Precipitating factors |
|---|---|
| Predisposing factors | Perpetuating (maintaining) factors (thoughts and beliefs, unhelpful behaviours and perceptions) |
| Protective factors | |

## References

21 Children's Workforce Development Council (CWDC). *The Common Assessment Framework for Children and Young People: a guide for practitioners*. CWDC: London, 2009.
22 Department of Health. *Effective Care Coordination in Mental Health Services: modernising the Care Programme Approach*. Department of Health: London, 1999.

## Further reading

Johnstone L and Dallos R. *Formulation in Psychology and Psychotherapy: making sense of people's problems*. Routledge: Hove, 2006.
McDougall T (ed.). *Child and Adolescent Mental Health Nursing*. Wiley-Blackwell: Oxford, 2006.

# Interventions in child and adolescent mental health

### Introduction

Nurses in Child and Adolescent Mental Health Services (CAMHS) usually adopt a holistic and eclectic approach when working with children and adolescents.

The core skill and underlying principle of all therapeutic models is the development of a therapeutic relationship.

Factors that influence the choice of model include:
- the developmental stage of the child
- the evidence base
- the qualifications and training of the nurse
- the preferences of the child or adolescent and their family.

### Core knowledge

This includes:
- child development.
- mental health problems that present in childhood and adolescence
- child protection and safeguarding policies and procedures
- risk factors and resilience factors:
  - *child risk factors*—genetics, low IQ, developmental delay, communication difficulties, physical illness, academic failure, low self-esteem
  - *child resilience factors*—self-esteem, autonomy, secure attachments, sociability
  - *family risk factors*—parental conflict, family breakdown, inconsistent discipline, rejection, abuse, failing to meet developmental needs, parental psychiatric illness, parental drug and alcohol misuse, parental criminality, death or relationship breakdown
  - *family resilience factors*—family compassion, warmth, minimal discord, good support.

### Core skills

These include:
- continuous risk assessment
- listening and attending
- communication and social skills
- observations of social interaction, play, mood, behaviour, sleep, and diet
- formulating—hypothesizing
- managing care collaboratively with the child or adolescent and their family
- partnership working with other services and agencies.

### Specialist skills

These include:
- *motivational interviewing*—a communication technique that promotes decision making and behaviour change

- *problem solving*—brainstorming the advantages and disadvantages of possible solutions, and implementing the best option
- *psychoeducation*—to understand and use the young person's strengths and resources to enable them to cope better with their presenting problems.

## Models of psychotherapy

- Behaviour therapy—based on social learning theories, helps young people and their families to change behaviours.
- Child psychodynamic psychotherapy—weekly sessions help children and adolescents to come to terms with complex emotional and relationship problems.
- Cognitive behavioural therapy—helps children and adolescents to understand the connections between their thoughts, feelings, and behaviours, in order to bring about change.
- Dialectic behaviour therapy—involves teaching life skills, such as tolerating distress, mindfulness, emotional regulation, interpersonal relationships, and finding a balance between change and acceptance.
- Solution-focused brief therapy—focuses on the present and the future, and helps young people to work towards their own goals, using questioning techniques such as the 'miracle question'.
- Systemic family therapy—skilled questioning and reflections help families to explore their interconnected system of relationships and discover ways to change.
- Multisystemic therapy—wider systems a re managed to ensure that the young person receives a consistent package of care. This approach is helpful for young people with severe conduct disorder, where education, youth justice, social services, and others are involved.

## Modes of delivery

- Creative therapies (drama, art, dance, and music)—help children and adolescents to express themselves and discover ways to change.
- Group therapy—provides support and an environment for change.
- Individual therapy.
- Intensive intervention—inpatient and day care facilities that are suitable for more serious and persistent mental health problems.
- Parenting training—based on social learning theories, this is structured, delivered on a sessional basis, and helps to improve parenting practices.
- Play therapy—helps children to recover through communication and play.
- Pharmacology—this should be used in accordance with NICE guidance; medication can be prescribed to children and adolescents in combination with other psychotherapy or talking therapies.

## Further reading

Department of Health. *National Service Framework for Children, Young People and Maternity Services*. Department of Health: London, 2004.
McDougall T (ed.). *Child and Adolescent Mental Health Nursing*. Wiley-Blackwell: Oxford, 2006.

# Chapter 5

# Violence

**Richard Whittington**

**Patrick Callaghan**

# Recognizing violence

Violence risk assessment has two main timescales for predicting the likelihood of imminent violence:
- short-term prediction (hours or minutes)
- long-term prediction (days, months, or years).

## Types of aggression

A useful distinction is between reactive ('hot', emotional) and proactive ('cold', instrumental) aggression, although there is much overlap between them.

*Reactive aggression* is a response to an identifiable, proximal trigger or provocation. It has the primary aim of harming the person or the object associated with the trigger, it is largely unplanned, and it is accompanied by signs of high levels of autonomic system arousal and loss of control.

*Proactive aggression* is a more planned response in the absence of immediate provocation or high levels of arousal. It has the primary aim of achieving a specific goal (e.g. escape or power) other than causing direct harm to the targeted person.

## Assessment of potential violence

This assessment relies both on close monitoring of the person's behaviour and on engaging with them from admission onward. It should take place in the context of an understanding of the person's background and personal triggers, and within a therapeutic relationship. The most useful predictor is the person's history of previous violence, and the triggers associated with such violence.

Much aggression in mental health services is reactive, occurring in response to perceived provocations. Behaviours that indicate angry arousal and potential loss of control in humans include:
- shouting
- glaring
- swearing
- verbal abuse
- verbal threats
- unclear or confused thinking
- intimidation
- use of the body (including intrusive gestures)
- restlessness.

Certain additional predictors are specifically linked to mental disorder, especially evidence of delusions or hallucinations with a violent content. The presence of these behaviours is associated with an elevated risk of imminent violence.

Each person has their own individual pattern of behaviour, and the presence of the behaviours listed does not necessarily indicate that violence is inevitable, nor does their absence automatically indicate that there is a low risk of imminent violence. Some acts of aggression occur following a period of withdrawal and silence. The key observation to be alert for is any rapid change in behaviour from the person's norm, and it is also important to be aware of current stressors or provocations.

## Instruments for assessing the risk of violence
- The Brøset Violence Checklist (BVC).
- The Violence Risk Appraisal Guide (VRAG).

## Further reading

Almvik R and Woods P. Short-term risk prediction: the Brøset Violence Checklist. *Journal of Psychiatric and Mental Health Nursing* 2003; **10**: 231–8.

Harris G, Rice M and Camillen J. Applying a forensic actuarial assessment (the Violence Risk Appraisal Guide) to non-forensic patients. *Journal of Interpersonal Violence* 2004; **19**: 1063–74.

# Preventing violence

Once the potential risk has been established, there is much that can be done to reduce the likelihood of violence occurring.

## Organizational level

At the organizational level, both the physical environment and the human environment can be improved (e.g. ward sightlines, the skill mix of staff, the staff–patient ratio). Training for staff and individualized risk assessment and activity programmes for patients can also be developed. A culture of service user collaboration and involvement should be fostered.

## Individual level

At the individual level, as soon as possible after admission the service user should be involved with the staff in identifying their own personal anger triggers and their preferred staff responses. This may be done using an advance directive (➜ Joint crisis plans for people with psychosis, p. 137).

## Preventative intervention

The interactional level becomes important once violence is judged to be imminent. Three main types of preventative intervention are available—enhanced observation and engagement, de-escalation, and preventative pharmacotherapy.

### Enhanced observation and engagement

General observation of inpatients can be stepped up to intermittent (15-minute) checks and observation, and then to 'within eyesight' and 'within arm's length' levels, as the risk escalates. Observation should involve active engagement of the observing staff with the service user at all times.

### De-escalation

De-escalation is a set of verbal and non-verbal skills used by staff to reduce the service user's level of angry arousal.

De-escalation skills include:
- establishing a rapport by demonstrating attentiveness, concern, and empathy
- reflection and active listening
- using open questions
- negotiation and encouraging a sense of cooperation
- modelling calmness.

De-escalation may include therapeutic limit setting and instructing, especially for proactive aggression, although this is likely to increase anger levels in the short term.

De-escalation techniques include:
- identifying the source of the person's anger
- explaining the reasons for the perceived provocations
- suggesting alternatives
- reminders of the time, place, and people involved in the interaction
- non-verbal indicators of interest, concern (e.g. head nodding), and personal calmness (e.g. relaxed posture).

Unnecessary proximity, touching, and a hectoring tone of voice should be avoided.

*Preventative pharmacotherapy*

This involves persuading (not coercing, although the line can be hard to draw) the service user to accept low levels of tranquillizing medication orally. Such medications include haloperidol, lorazepam, olanzapine, and risperidone.

## Further reading

Cowin L et al. De-escalating aggression and violence in the mental health setting. *International Journal of Mental Health Nursing* 2003; **12**: 64–73.

National Institute for Health and Care Excellence (NICE). *Violence: the short-term management of disturbed/violent behaviour in in-patient psychiatric settings and emergency departments*. CG25. NICE: London, 2005.

# Therapeutic management of violence

Effective prediction and prevention will help to avoid most, but not all, incidents developing into overt violence. If prevention is judged to be failing, and the only alternative available is to manage the threat, therapeutic management may be used. This is likely to include some degree of coercion. Restrictive interventions should only be used as a last resort. For DH guidance on minimizing the use of restrictive interventions please refer to the following link ℘ https://www.gov.uk/government/publications/positive-and-proactive-care-reducing-restrictive-interventions

## Principles

The level of coercion used must be proportional to the threat presented by the person, and any coercion should be ended as soon as possible, without compromising safety. Potential non-coercive alternatives should always be considered.

Explicit policies that provide guidance on the use of coercive interventions and recording mechanisms must be in place. Positive engagement and de-escalation activities (➲ Preventing violence, p. 154) must continue alongside coercive interventions, but the potential for negotiation is much reduced at this stage.

There are three main techniques for the therapeutic management of violence—physical restraint, seclusion, and rapid tranquillization.

## Physical (manual) restraint

Physical restraint is used for the immediate emergency management of violence. It involves holding the person and preventing their movement. A standing position should be maintained if at all possible, as restraint on the floor can be highly dangerous, and direct pressure on certain parts of the body (e.g. the thorax) can be fatal. A team member should be responsible for supporting the person's head and neck, ensuring that their airway and breathing are not compromised, and monitoring vital signs.

## Seclusion

Seclusion involves the enforced segregation of a person in a bare room or an area separate from the ward community. The exit from this room is either locked or blocked by allocated staff. Observation and engagement should be maintained throughout the seclusion period.

Many authorities view seclusion as the most anti-therapeutic of the coercive interventions, and active steps to police it and to reduce its use are being taken worldwide. Some argue for mechanical restraint as an acceptable alternative.

## Rapid tranquillization

This involves the administration of tranquillizing medication, which may have to be done intramuscularly or intravenously while the person is held under restraint. Negotiated acceptance of oral medication may be possible as an alternative, and should be considered on the principle of least coercive care. Medications that are given include haloperidol and lorazepam. Observation and, where possible, engagement should be maintained throughout the sedation period.

Throughout this process of managing violence, the needs of other service users should be considered by allocating at least one staff member to support them if necessary.

## Further reading

National Institute for Health and Care Excellence (NICE). *Violence: the short-term management of disturbed/violent behaviour in in-patient psychiatric settings and emergency departments.* CG25. NICE: London, 2005.

Sailas E and Wahlbeck K. Restraint and seclusion in psychiatric inpatient wards. *Current Opinion in Psychiatry* 2005; **18**: 555–9.

# Post-violence incident analysis and management

Once the immediate crisis has been resolved, and a safe environment has been restored, the aftermath of a violent incident must be managed, and this includes efforts to learn from the experience. All service users and staff who were directly involved in or witnessed the incident should be considered.

The first priority is to assess and manage any physical injury sustained by any person as a result of the incident. Physical injury may be treated locally or may require referral to an emergency department.

The second priority is to assess and minimize the psychological distress of those staff and service users who were directly or indirectly involved in the incident. Immediate reassurance and explanations should be provided as appropriate.

## Report or post-incident review

### Report

A brief, structured report on all violent incidents should be made by the lead person involved, as soon as possible after the incident. This report should follow a template that is used throughout the organization, and could be based on widely used forms, such as the Staff Observation of Aggression Scale–Revised (SOAS-R).[1] Electronic reporting will expedite communication and review.

### Post-incident review

This is more formal than a report. It involves staff, service users, and others as appropriate, and should be conducted within 72 hours after the incident. It aims to identify individual support needs and to inform future practice.

Those identified as experiencing significant distress as a result of the incident may require sickness absence, and a phased, supported return to work with service users, over a period of 1–2 weeks or longer.

Lessons for improved practice are learned through incident analysis. This involves discussion of the relevant warning signs and triggers that preceded the incident, and the effectiveness of any physical and psychological techniques that were used to manage the violence. The role of the environment in the incident should also be considered. The tone of the post-incident review should be neutral and non-blaming, and where possible the review should be conducted by someone who was not directly involved.

A collaborative review with the relevant service user is also recommended, to minimize damage to the therapeutic relationship. Action points identified from the review should be incorporated into individual care plans and unit policies. If incidents occur regularly, teams should consider a weekly or monthly review to identify any common patterns, and should act to incorporate these into care plans and risk assessments for individual service users.

*Institutional post-incident reviews* by senior staff should also be conducted regularly. These are based on the incident reports, and aim to identify patterns across units and to develop an action plan.

## Reference

1 Nijman HLI, Palmstierna T, Almvik R and Stolker JJ. Fifteen years of research with the Staff Observation Aggression Scale: a review. *Acta Psychiatrica Scandinavica* 2005; **111**: 12–21.

## Further reading

Flannery RB Jr. The Assaulted Staff Action Program (ASAP): ten year empirical support for critical incident stress management (CISM). *International Journal of Emergency Mental Health* 2001; **3**: 5–10.

# Possibilities and pitfalls in violence risk assessment

### Introduction

Despite progress in the care and treatment of people with mental health problems, the prevalence of violent incidents—that is, verbal or physical aggression directed at self or others—remains high in many parts of the world. Risk assessment is a widely used method of seeking to predict future violence with a view to preventing or minimizing the occurrence of violence and managing people whose behaviour is deemed harmful[2,3] (see Table 5.1). This approach is referred to as the assessment–prediction–intervention model.[3] Risk assessment generally takes two forms—actuarial measures and structured clinical judgement.

### Actuarial measures

These are specially developed scales that offer the possibility of making accurate risk predictions. Actuarial measures of risk typically contain items that assess an individual's violence history, diagnosis, personality, and social support. Using these measures an assessor will compute a score that invariably allows the risk level to be categorized as low, moderate, or high.

**Table 5.1** Possibilities and pitfalls associated with violence risk assessment

| Possibilities | Pitfalls |
| --- | --- |
| Reductions in violence | There is little evidence that risk assessments reduce violence |
| Increased accuracy of risk predictions | People deemed at low risk may not get access to mental health care |
| Actuarial measures allow prediction of the number of people that need to be treated in order to prevent at least one violent incident | Calculations derived from actuarial measures are correlations; they do not allow cause-and-effect conclusions |
| Clinicians can develop interventions to reduce or prevent violence | The most effective and evidence-based interventions have little to do with risk assessments |
| Mental health practitioners with the powers to detain people involuntarily may benefit from access to the best available risk assessment measures | Detention on the grounds of risk discriminates against people who have a mental disorder, and this situation should sit uneasily in democratic societies with strong civil libertarian principles enshrined in law |
| | The efficacy of risk assessment measures may depend on the type of risk that is being assessed (i.e. they have little generic value) |

## Structured clinical judgement

This is a process whereby an assessor uses their clinical judgement to decide on the level of risk, aided where necessary by a rating scale.

## References

2  Singh JP, Grann M and Fazel S. A comparative study of violence risk assessment tolls: a systematic review and meta-regression analysis of 68 studies involving 25,980 participants. *Clinical Psychology Review* 2011; **31**: 499–513.

3  Yang M, Wong SCP and Coid J. The efficacy of violence prediction: a meta-analytic comparison of nine risk assessment tools. *Psychological Bulletin* 2010; **136**: 740–67.

## Further reading

Callaghan P. Possibilities and pitfalls in violence risk assessment and management. In: I Needham et al. (eds) *Proceedings of the 7th European Congress on Violence in Clinical Psychiatry*, Prague, 19–22 October 2009. p. 33.

# Chapter 6

# Risk

**Patrick Callaghan**

# Risk assessment: violence

Risk is the likelihood of behaviour that may be harmful or beneficial to one-self or to others. Risk assessment involves analysing the potential outcomes of this behaviour, and risk management involves devising a care plan to minimize harmful behaviour and maximize beneficial behaviour.

## Prevalence of violence in the UK
- There were 61,571 violent incidents in the NHS in 2012–2013.[1]
- Mental health settings accounted for 43,699 of these incidents.
- In mental health services there were 210 assaults per staff member.

## Consequences of violence
- Sickness from work.
- Physical injury, which is sometimes serious.
- Post-traumatic stress disorder (PTSD).
- A profound sense of alienation.
- Persistent fear.

## Demographic predictors of violence
- Previous history of violence to people or property.
- History of misuse of substances or alcohol.
- Previous expression of intent to harm others.
- Evidence of rootlessness or social restlessness.
- Previous dangerous or impulsive acts.
- Previous use of weapons.
- Denial of previous dangerous acts.
- Verbal threats of violence.

## Clinical predictors of violence
- Misuse of drugs or alcohol.
- Drug effects (e.g. disinhibition).
- Delusions or hallucinations focused on a particular person.
- Command hallucinations (i.e. responding to voices commanding one to perform a certain act).
- Preoccupation with violent fantasy.
- Delusions of control.
- Agitation, excitement, overt hostility, or suspicion.
- Poor collaboration with suggested treatments.
- Organic dysfunction (e.g. forms of dementia).

## Situational predictors of violence
- Extent of social support.
- Immediate availability of potential weapon.
- Relationship to victim.
- Access to potential victim.
- Staff setting limits on service users.
- Staff attitudes.

## Antecedents and warning signs

- Tense and angry facial expression.
- Increased or prolonged restlessness.
- General overarousal.
- Increased volume of speech.
- Erratic movements.
- Prolonged eye contact.
- Discontentment, refusal to communicate, withdrawal, fear, or irritation.
- Unclear thought processes and poor concentration.
- Delusions or hallucinations with violent content.
- Verbal threats or gestures.
- Reporting anger or violent feelings.
- Replicating previous behaviour that led to violence.

## Risk assessment

Assessment should:
- be regular and comprehensive
- involve an assessment of staff attitudes, situations, and organizational and environmental factors linked to violence
- include a structured and sensitive interview with the service user, to focus on triggers, early warning signs, and other vulnerabilities
- avoid negative assumptions based on ethnicity
- involve a multidisciplinary approach
- assess and record service users' preferences for managing violence.

## Actuarial measures used in risk assessment

- Psychopathy Checklist–Revised (PCL-R).
- Violence Risk Appraisal Guide (VRAG).
- Historical, Clinical, Risk Management 20-item scale (HCR-20).
- Dangerous Behaviour Rating Scale (DBRS).

## Reference

1 NHS Business Services Authority. *2012–13 Figures Released for Reported Physical Assaults on NHS Staff.* ℘ www.nhsbsa.nhs.uk/4380.aspx

## Further reading

Moghan S. *Clinical Risk Management: a clinical tool and practitioner manual.* The Sainsbury Centre for Mental Health: London, 2000.

National Institute for Health and Care Excellence (NICE). *Violence: the short-term management of disturbed/violent behaviour in in-patient psychiatric settings and emergency departments.* CG25. NICE: London, 2005.

NHS Protect report ℘ http://www.nhsbsa.nhs.uk/Documents/SecurityManagement/NHS_Protect_Annual_Report_2013-14.pdf

# Risk assessment: suicide

## Introduction

Risk is the likelihood of behaviour that may be harmful or beneficial to one-self or to others. Risk assessment involves analysing the potential outcomes of this behaviour, and risk management involves devising a care plan to minimize harmful behaviour and maximize beneficial behaviour (see Table 6.1). Suicide remains a major public health concern. In the UK there are around 5000 suicides each year, 75% of which are in men, and suicide is the second most frequent cause of death in men under 35 years of age. Around 90% of people who die by suicide have a mental disorder, most commonly depression (60% of cases). Mental health nurses working in a range of settings are likely to encounter people at risk of suicide. It is estimated that 50% of suicides will have had contact with a GP 3 months prior to their death, 40% will have had such contact 1 month before death, and 20% in the week before death.[2]

## Risk factors for suicide

*Assessing suicide risk*[2]

Six key questions are indicated when assessing a person's suicide risk:
- Are they feeling hopeless, or that life is not worth living?
- Have they made plans to end their life?
- Have they told anyone about it?
- Have they carried out any acts in anticipation of death (e.g. putting their affairs in order)?

Table 6.1 Risk factors for suicide

| Risk factors specific to depression | Other risk factors | Possible protective factors |
|---|---|---|
| Family history of mental disorder | Family history of suicide or self-harm | Social support |
| History of previous attempts (including self-harm) | Physical illness (especially if recently diagnosed or chronic and painful) | Religious belief |
| Severe depression | | Being responsible for children (especially young children) |
| Anxiety | Exposure to suicidal behaviour of others | |
| Feelings of hopelessness | Recent discharge from psychiatric inpatient care | |
| Personality disorder | Access to potentially lethal means of self-harm or suicide | |
| Alcohol and/or drug use | | |
| Male gender | | |

- Do they have the means for a suicidal act (i.e. do they have access to pills, firearms, insecticides, etc.)?
- Is there any available support (family, friends, carers)?

*Managing suicide risk²*
- Assess the risk.
- Share the findings of the risk assessment with other members of the care team.
- Share your concerns with the person who is being assessed.
- Treat the underlying depression as soon as possible.
- Provide contact details of team members, including out-of-hours contact numbers.
- Alert the administrative staff so that they can prioritize calls from people who may be at high risk.

*The government's approach to suicide prevention in England³*
- Reduce the suicide risk in high-risk groups.
- Tailor approaches to improve mental health in specific groups.
- Reduce access to the means of suicide.
- Provide better information and support to those who have been bereaved or affected by suicide.
- Support the media in delivering sensitive approaches to suicide and suicidal behaviour.
- Support research, data collection, and monitoring.
- Make it a priority both locally and nationally.

## References
2 Centre for Suicide Research. *Assessment of Suicide Risk in People with Depression*. Available at ♂ http://cebmh.warne.ox.ac.uk/csr/Clinical_guide_assessing_suicide_risk.pdf
3 Department of Health. *Preventing Suicide in England: a cross-government outcomes strategy to save lives*. Department of Health: London, 2012.

## Further reading
National Institute for Health and Care Excellence (NICE). *Self-Harm: the short-term physical and psychological management and secondary prevention of self-harm in primary and secondary care*. CG16. NICE: London, 2004.

# Risk assessment: abuse

Risk is the likelihood of behaviour that may be harmful or beneficial to one-self or to others. Risk assessment involves analysing the potential outcomes of this behaviour, and risk management involves devising a care plan to minimize harmful behaviour and maximize beneficial behaviour.

## Types of abuse

- *Physical*—includes punching, pushing, and hitting.
- *Sexual*—includes rape, sexual assault, and sexual acts performed without consent or where consent could not be given.
- *Psychological*—includes emotional abuse, threats, and humiliation.
- *Financial*—includes theft, fraud, and exploitation.
- *Neglect*—includes ignoring needs and withholding the necessities of life.
- *Discrimination*—includes racism, sexism, ageism, and harassment.
- *Institutional*—includes poor professional service and ill treatment.

## Risk factors associated with abuse

For all types of abuse the risk factors are unequal power, social isolation, and a vulnerable family history of violence and abuse.

Other risk factors include:
- *Physical abuse*—long delays in reporting injuries, unexplained bruises, misuse of medication.
- *Sexual abuse*—overly sexual conversations and behaviour.
- *Psychological abuse*—ambivalence about the carer, unexplained paranoia, passivity, or resignation.
- *Financial abuse*—unusual account activity, excessive gifts to carers.
- *Neglect*—person left alone in an unsafe environment, refusal of access to visitors or callers, violation of privacy and dignity.
- *Rights violation*—coercion, refusal of access to visitors or callers, lack of respect, lack of attention to personal hygiene.
- *Institutional*—rigid routines, poor standards of cleanliness, 'batch' care.

## Risk assessment

- Conduct an assessment interview.
- Perform a mental state assessment.
- Take a history of abuse incidents.
- Assess specific indicators of abuse (see paragraph above).
- Assess for any discrepancy between what is reported and what is observed.
- Assess for any discrepancy between verbal and non-verbal cues.
- Assess coping potential and availability of social support.

## Assessment of the seriousness of abuse

This should include:
- the vulnerability of the individual
- the nature and extent of the abuse
- the length of time for which the abuse has been occurring
- the impact on the individual
- repeated or increasingly serious acts of abuse
- the intent of the person alleged to be responsible for the abuse.

## Management of abuse

- Ensure the safety of the victim.
- Discuss concerns with colleagues or the multidisciplinary team.
- Make appropriate referrals to the care management team, the social services team, and the police/registration inspection unit.
- Consider what treatment or therapy is appropriate.
- Ensure any necessary modification in the way that services are provided.
- Support the individual through any appropriate action that they take to seek justice or redress.
- Use stress management techniques.
- Encourage the vulnerable person to remain active and independent, and to maintain social contacts.
- Work with the person's significant others to discuss the best forms of support or aftercare.

## Further reading

Department of Health. *Domestic Violence: a resources manual for health care professionals*. Department of Health: London, 2000.

Oxleas Mental Health Trust. *A Guide to the Assessment and Management of Risk*. Oxleas Mental Health Trust: London, 2002. pp. 37–59.

# Risk assessment: self-neglect

Risk is the likelihood of behaviour that may be harmful or beneficial to oneself or to others. Risk assessment involves analysing the potential outcomes of this behaviour, and risk management involves devising a care plan to minimize harmful behaviour and maximize beneficial behaviour (see Table 6.2).

### Risk factors to consider during assessment for self-neglect

- Hygiene.
- Diet.
- Physical health.
- Medication.
- Substance misuse.
- Adequacy of clothing.
- Capacity to self-care.
- Capacity to seek help.
- Adequacy of accommodation.
- Household safety.
- Basic household amenities.
- Infestation.
- Financial situation.

Table 6.2 Risk factors for self-neglect

| Higher risk | Lower risk |
| --- | --- |
| Female | Male |
| Living alone | Living with others |
| Mental illness: dementia, psychosis | Good health |
| Single, widowed, or separated | Married or in stable relationship |
| Substance misuse | No substance misuse |
| Poor housing | Satisfactory accommodation |
| Loss of significant other | No loss of significant other |
| Poor physical health | No cognitive or sensory impairments |
| Sensory and cognitive impairments | |
| Unable to seek help | Living with competent carers |
| Vulnerable to exploitation | Able to seek help |

### Risk assessment

- Take a history—assess awareness of illness or vulnerability, capacity to identify, understand, and manage risks, engagement with treatment or services, and premorbid personality.
- Discover the view of significant others—note any expressions of concern.
- Assess ideation and mental state—capacity to make decisions and think about ways to manage risks, willingness to accept support, present state examination.
- Assess intent—the degree of intent to engage in a risky behaviour.

- Assess planning—whether the person has made any plans to engage in risky behaviour.
- Assess awareness of risk—the person's view of the problem.
- Assess the benefits versus the harms of risky behaviour.

## Deciding on the nature and severity of the risk

1. How serious is the risk?
2. Is the risk specific or general?
3. How immediate is the risk?
4. How volatile is the risk?
5. Are circumstances likely to arise that will increase the risk?
6. What specific treatment and management plan can best reduce the risk?

## Management

- The Care Programme Approach (CPA; ➋ Assessment frameworks and tools, p. 146) is important. Plan care with the service user and their significant others.
- Identification of antecedents of self-neglect behaviour (see earlier in this topic).
- Increased monitoring.
- Access to supported housing.
- Use of Section 117 if necessary.
- Environmental health assessment and treatment of property if necessary.

## Further reading

Johnson J and Adams J. Self-neglect in later life. *Health and Social Care in the Community* 1996; 4: 226–33.

Oxleas Mental Health Trust. *A Guide to the Assessment and Management of Risk*. Oxleas Mental Health Trust: London, 2002. pp. 23–35.

# Risk assessment: falls

Risk is the likelihood of behaviour that may be harmful or beneficial to one-self or to others. Risk assessment involves analysing the potential outcomes of this behaviour, and risk management involves devising a care plan to minimize harmful behaviour and maximize beneficial behaviour.

## General areas to cover in the assessment

- Risk factors (see Table 6.3).
- History.
- Physical health.
- Environmental factors.
- Information from relatives and carers.
- Ideation/mental state.
- Intent.
- Planning.
- The person's awareness of risk.
- Benefits and harms associated with risk.
- Formulation.

## Risk assessment of falls

- Assess current symptoms.
- Take a history of previous falls, noting in particular: Location, Activity, Time, Trauma. Assess the views of significant others.
- Assess ideation and mental state—awareness of illness, vulnerability, and capacity to make decisions.
- Assess awareness of risk.
- Consider the benefits and harms associated with risk.
- Identification of falls history.
- Assess gait, balance, mobility, and muscle weakness.
- Assess osteoporosis risk.
- Assess the person's perceived functional ability, and their fear of falling.
- Assess visual impairment.
- Assess cognitive impairment and perform a neurological examination.
- Assess urinary incontinence.
- Assess home hazards.
- Conduct a cardiovascular examination and review.

## Multifactorial management

- Strength and balance training.
- Home hazard assessment and intervention.
- Vision assessment and referral for treatment if necessary.
- Medication review with modification or withdrawal.
- Cardiac pacing.
- Provide oral and written information for users and significant others about recommended measures to prevent further falls, and how to cope in the event of a fall.

## Rating scales for assessment of falls risk

- Falls Risk Assessment Scale for the Elderly (FRASE).
- St Thomas's Risk Assessment Tool in Falling Elderly Inpatients (STRATIFY).

**Table 6.3** Risk factors for falls

| Variable | Higher risk | Lower risk |
|---|---|---|
| Age | Older | Younger |
| Past history | Falling incidents in past 12 months | No history of falls |
| Physical status | Medical problems, especially circulatory ones | Few or no medical problems |
| Environment | Hazardous | Not hazardous |
| Mental state | Sensory and cognitive impairment | No sensory or cognitive impairment |
| Medication | Combinations that affect balance | Combinations that do not affect balance |
| Mobility | Poor, with gait and balance problems | No problems |

## Further reading

National Institute for Health and Care Excellence (NICE). *Falls: assessment and prevention of falls in older people.* CG161. NICE: London, 2013.

Oxleas Mental Health Trust. *A Guide to the Assessment and Management of Risk.* Oxleas Mental Health Trust: London, 2002. pp. 107–17.

# Risk assessment: fire

Risk is the likelihood of behaviour that may be harmful or beneficial to one-self or to others. Risk assessment involves analysing the potential outcomes of this behaviour, and risk management involves devising a care plan to mini-mize harmful behaviour and maximize beneficial behaviour.

## Areas to cover in the assessment

- Risk factors (see Table 6.4).
- History.
- Information from relatives and carers.
- Ideation and mental state.
- Intent.
- Planning.
- The person's awareness of risk.
- The benefits and harms associated with risk.
- Formulation.

## Risk assessment

- Assess the person. Do they exhibit risk factors? Do they exhibit safety awareness?
- Assess the environment. Is there potential fuel for fires? Is there a fire-alerting system? Is there a potential fire escape, and is the person able to use it?
- Consider other people. Is there a potential risk to others?

## Assessment of the nature of previous fire setting

- *Timing*. How recent was the risk or behaviour?
- *Severity*.
- *Frequency*. Was it an isolated incident, or does it happen frequently?
- *Pattern*. Is there a common pattern to the type of incident or the context in which it occurs?

## Management of the risk of fire setting

- Arrange further specialist assessment.
- Arrange admission to hospital if arson intent is present.
- Make the person's environment safer.
- Provide fire-alerting devices.
- Ensure that the person is supervised during procedures that may be risky, such as cooking, smoking, or using appliances.

**Table 6.4** Risk factors for fire setting

| Variable | Higher risk | Lower risk |
| --- | --- | --- |
| Past history of arson | Past history, especially if recent, or younger age at first fire setting | No history |
| Past history of accidental fire setting | Past history, especially if recent | No history |
| Use of potential sources of fire | Poor safety awareness<br>Smoker<br>Unsafe appliances<br>Unsafe behaviour (e.g. leaving cooking pans unattended, leaving gas on, overloading electric circuits) | Good safety awareness<br>Non-smoker<br>Safe appliances<br>Safe behaviour |
| Environment | Potential fuel for fire<br>No fire-alerting system<br>Electrical cords under furniture or carpeting | Little potential fuel for fire<br>Fire-alerting system (e.g. working smoke alarm) |
| Learning disability | Mild learning disability with poor social and communication skills | Severe learning disability |

## Further reading

Oxleas Mental Health Trust. *A Guide to the Assessment and Management of Risk*. Oxleas Mental Health Trust: London, 2002. pp. 119–230.

# Common mental disorders

## Understanding mental illness

Mental illness refers collectively to all diagnosable mental disorders characterized by alterations in thinking, mood, or behaviour, or a combination of these, mediated by the brain and associated with distress and impaired functioning. There have been concerted efforts to develop systems of classification of mental illness that would be suitable for use across different cultures. Two classification systems are used:

• The *Diagnostic and Statistical Manual of Mental Disorders*, Fifth Edition (DSM-5).[1]
• The *International Statistical Classification of Diseases and Related Health Problems*, Tenth Revision (ICD-10)—this is the classification system used primarily in the UK.[2]

Both of these systems have gone some way toward providing uniformity and consistency with regard to the diagnosis and classification of mental illness. These classification systems do have an important place, as they help to distinguish the severely ill from the moderately or mildly ill. The absence of such systems would hamper the ability to plan services, evaluate treatments or interventions, or evaluate the effectiveness of preventative strategies.[3]

We may all experience one or more of the symptoms described in either of these classification systems at some point in our life. It is unhelpful, meaningless, and stigmatizing to have personal distress labelled in such a manner that people respond to the label rather than to the individual. This is demonstrated by the comparison in Table 7.1.

It is more important to understand the experience of the person who is living with mental health problems than to attempt to understand mental illness per se.

### Note:

Comorbidity refers to the existence of two or more illnesses in the same individual.

Serious mental illness (SMI) refers to an illness that is long-lasting and severely interferes with a person's ability to participate in life activities.

**Table 7.1** Comparison of the psychosocial and biomedical perspectives

| Criteria | Psychosocial perspective | Biomedical perspective |
|---|---|---|
| Cause of illness | Behaviour, beliefs, poverty, coping mechanisms, relationships, childhood trauma | Genetics, brain injury, viral or bacterial infection, birth trauma, neurotransmitter imbalance |
| Responsibility for illness | Individual, social, political, environmental, and economic factors | External forces that cause internal change |
| Treatment of illness | Holistic approach: change in beliefs, coping style, economic status, relationships | Medication or other medical intervention, surgery, electroconvulsive therapy |
| Responsibility for treatment | Individual, family, significant other, support networks | The doctor and other professionals involved in collaboration with the individual |
| Relationship between mental health and illness | Both exist on a continuum, with varying degrees of mental health and mental illness | Dichotomous—the person is either healthy or ill |
| Relationship between mind and body | The mind and body are mutually interdependent | The mind and body function independently of one another |
| Role in health and illness | Psychosocial factors contribute to an individual's mental health status | Illness has psychosocial consequences, not causes |

### References

1 American Psychiatric Association. *Diagnostic and Statistical Manual of Mental Disorders*, Fifth Edition (DSM-5). American Psychiatric Publishing: Arlington, VA, 2013.
2 World Health Organization. *International Classification of Mental and Behavioural Disorders*, Tenth Revision (ICD-10). World Health Organization: Geneva, 1992.
3 Newton J. *Preventing Mental Illness*. Routledge: London, 1988.

# *Diagnostic and Statistical Manual of Mental Disorders*, Fifth Edition (DSM-5)

## Introduction

Differences in defining and describing mental illness and mental health led to a concerted effort by psychiatrists to develop systems for classifying mental illness that would be relevant for use across cultures and which could be used by clinicians to detect, diagnose, and treat mental illness. The two classification systems used are the *Diagnostic and Statistical Manual of Mental Disorders,* Fifth Edition (DSM-5), published by the American Psychiatric Association (APA) in 2013, and the *International Classification of Mental and Behavioural Disorders,* now in its tenth revision (ICD-10), published by the World Health Organization in 1992.

DSM was first published in 1959, primarily to provide the US military with a guide on the diagnoses of service personnel. DSM seeks to provide psychiatrists with a definitive list of all recognized mental health conditions, describing their clinical features, and is designed to enable psychiatrists to make accurate diagnoses. The DSM classification system is highly controversial, and the main arguments for and against it are outlined in Table 7.2. Please refer to the Further reading list at the end of this section for more detailed critiques of the arguments.

**Table 7.2** Arguments for and against DSM-5

| Arguments for DSM-5 | Arguments against DSM-5 |
| --- | --- |
| • Enables more accurate diagnoses that help people to access appropriate treatment, care, services, and benefits | • Lack of empirical validity for many of the conditions listed |
| • Mental disorder is often uncertain, and it helps to have a diagnostic guide to which people can refer for information | • Over-'medicalizing' of mental health |
| • The best available method of classifying mental disorder | • Focus on conditions rather than on people |
| • Includes a large amount of practical knowledge in a useful format | • Cannot reasonably account for the individual differences in the way that people experience different conditions |
| | • Takes a 'top-down' approach in which people are made to fit conditions |
| | • Overly strong influence of the pharmaceutical industry as evidenced by the DSM-5 taskforce membership |
| | • Lack of prognostic value |

## Changes from DSM-IV-TR to DSM-5

Each reiteration of DSM inevitably involves changes in the number of conditions included, and the features of different conditions. The APA has published a detailed description of the changes to DSM-5 compared with the previous edition. These details can be accessed from the following website: ℰ www. ldaofky.org/changes-from-dsm-iv-tr--to-dsm-5%5B1%5D.pdf

Classification systems such as DSM-5 have gone some way toward redressing some of the chaos that existed in previous attempts to classify mental disorders in a manner that was satisfactory, valid, and had cross-cultural relevance. However, they have been criticized for their 'failure to represent the diversity of human experiences of distress',[4] and they often reflect commercial interests, are individualistic, reflect dominant conceptions of the 'Western' self, are social constructions, and lack empirical validity. These systems fail to account for the influences of race, identity, gender, class, and social power in people's experiences of distress. In short, attempts to classify mental illness are futile, unhelpful, and contribute little to alleviating people's distress. However, Newton[5] has argued that such classification systems help to distinguish the ill from the moderately or mildly ill. The absence of such systems, she maintains, would hamper our ability to plan services, evaluate the success of treatment and rehabilitation, or assess the effectiveness of preventive strategies.

## References

4 Parker I et al. *Deconstructing Psychopathology*. London: Sage, 1995.
5 Newton J. *Preventing Mental Illness*. London: Routledge, 1988.

## Further reading

American Psychiatric Association. *DSM-5: Frequently Asked Questions*. American Psychiatric Publishing: Arlington, VA, 2012. ℰ www.dsm5.org/about/pages/faq.aspx
American Psychiatric Association. *Highlights of Changes from DSM-IV-TR to DSM-5*. American Psychiatric Publishing: Arlington, VA, 2012. ℰ www.dsm5.org/Documents/changes%20 from%20dsm-iv-tr%20to%20dsm-5.pdf
British Psychological Society. *Response to the American Psychiatric Association DSM-5 Development*. British Psychological Society: London, 2011. ℰ http://apps.bps.org.uk/_publicationfiles/ consultation-responses/DSM-5%202011%20-%20BPS%20response.pdf
Frances AJ. *DSM 5 is Guide not Bible—Ignore its Ten Worst Changes*. ℰ www.psychologytoday.com/ blog/dsm5-in-distress/201212/dsm-5-is-guide-not-bible-ignore-its-ten-worst-changes
Frances AJ. *Last Plea to DSM 5: Save Grief From the Drug Companies*. ℰ https://www.psychology-today.com/blog/dsm5-in-distress/201301/last-plea-dsm-5-save-grief-the-drug-companies
Frances AJ and Widiger T. Psychiatric diagnosis: lessons from the DSM-IV past and cautions for the DSM-5 future. *Annual Review of Clinical Psychology* 2012; **8**: 109–30.
iPetitions. *Open Letter to the DSM-5*. ℰ www.ipetitions.com/petition/dsm5/
World Health Organization. *The ICD-10 Classification of Mental and Behavioural Disorders: clinical descriptions and diagnostic guidelines*. Geneva: World Health Organization, 1992.

# Anorexia nervosa

Anorexia nervosa is a condition in which there is a marked distortion of body image, low body weight, and weight loss behaviours (see Table 7.3). There is a mortality rate of 10–15% (two-thirds of deaths are due to physical complications and one-third due to suicide).

## Incidence

Around 0.5% of adolescent girls and young women develop anorexia nervosa. There is a male:female ratio of 1:10. There is an equal distribution across the social classes, with predominantly upper- and middle-class people seeking treatment.

## Criteria

- Low body weight—15% below normal for age, height, and body frame.
- Self-induced weight loss—by vomiting, purging, excessive exercise, use of appetite suppressants and laxatives.
- Body image distortion—dread of fatness, imposed low body weight threshold.
- Endocrine disorders—involving the hypothalamus, pituitary, or adrenal glands.
- Amenorrhoea, reduced sexual interest or impotence, small body frame, altered thyroid function.
- Delayed puberty (if the onset is prior to puberty).

**Table 7.3** Symptoms and signs of anorexia nervosa

| Mental health symptoms | Physical health symptoms | Common physical signs |
|---|---|---|
| Decreased concentration | General health concerns | Loss of muscle mass |
| Poor memory | Amenorrhoea | Dry skin |
| Irritability | Cold hands and feet | Brittle hair and nails |
| Depression | Weight loss | Anaemia |
| Low self-esteem | Constipation | Calluses on finger joints |
| Loss of appetite | Hair loss | Fine downy body hair |
| Reduced energy | Headaches | Eroded tooth enamel |
| Insomnia | Fainting or dizziness | Hypotension |
| Loss of libido | Lethargy | Bradycardia |
| Social withdrawal | Pale skin | Atrophy of the breasts |
| Obsessiveness about food | | Swollen tender abdomen |
| Reduced decision making | | Loss of sensation in the extremities |

## Aetiology

- Genetic—6–10% of female siblings develop the condition.
- Life events—*physical or sexual abuse can be risk factors.*
- Psychodynamic:
  - Family relationships may be rigid, overprotective, with weak parental boundaries, and lack of conflict resolution.
  - Individual—disturbed body image due to dietary problems in early life, parents' preoccupation with food, and lack of sense of identity.
  - Analytical—regression to childhood, fixation on the oral stage, and avoidance of problems in adolescence.

## Prognosis

- If untreated, this condition has one of the highest mortality rates of any mental health disorder.
- If treated, one-third of patients make a full recovery, one-third make a partial recovery, and one-third have chronic problems.
- Most cases are treated as outpatients, with a combined approach including:
  - Pharmacological treatment—antidepressants, medication to stimulate appetite.
  - Psychological therapy—family therapy (may be effective if early onset). Individual therapy, such as CBT—may improve long-term outcomes.
  - Education—nutritional and self-help manuals.
- Hospital admission should only be considered if there are serious medical problems. Compulsory admission may be required—feeding is regarded as treatment. Ethical issues have to be considered with regard to a person's right to die and their right to treatment.
- Poor prognostic factors include chronic illness, late age of onset, bulimic features, anxiety when eating with others, excessive weight loss, poor childhood social adjustment, poor parental relationships, and male gender.

➔ People with anorexia nervosa, p. 90.

## Further reading

Duker M and Slade R. *Anorexia Nervosa and Bulimia*, 2nd edn. Open University Press: Buckingham, 2002.
Eivors A and Nesbitts S. *Hunger for Understanding: a workbook for helping young people to understand and overcome anorexia nervosa.* John Wiley & Sons: Chichester, 2005.

# Bulimia nervosa

Bulimia nervosa is a condition characterized by recurrent episodes of binge eating, combined with compensatory behaviours and overvalued ideas about ideal body shape and weight. Body weight may be normal, although there is often a past history of anorexia nervosa (30–50% of cases).

## Incidence

Around 1–1.5% of women develop bulimia nervosa, with onset during mid adolescence, and presentation in the early twenties.

## Aetiology

The aetiology is similar to that of anorexia nervosa. There is also evidence for associated personal or family history of affective disorder and/or substance misuse.

## Diagnostic criteria

- Persistent preoccupation with eating.
- Irresistible craving for food.
- Episodes of overeating (bingeing).
- Attempts to counter the fattening effects of food with self-induced vomiting, purgative abuse, periods of starvation, or use of appetite suppressants and laxatives.
- Morbid dread of fatness, with an imposed low body weight threshold.

## Physical signs

- May be similar to those of anorexia nervosa, but may be less severe.
- Specific problems related to purging (laxative abuse) include:
  - arrhythmias
  - cardiac failure (with sudden death)
  - electrolyte disturbance due to laxatives or vomiting
  - oesophageal erosion due to excessive vomiting
  - oesophageal and gastric perforation
  - gastric and duodenal ulcers
  - pancreatitis
  - constipation and/or steatorrhoea
  - dental erosions
  - leucopenia and lymphocytosis.

## Treatment

- General principles:
  - Usually managed as an outpatient.
  - Admission is generally only for suicidality, physical problems, or pregnancy.
  - Combined treatment approaches improve the outcome.
- Medication—there is evidence for the effectiveness of high-dose antidepressants as long-term treatment.

- Psychotherapy:
  - The best evidence is for CBT.
  - Interpersonal therapy is effective in the long term, but takes longer to become effective.
  - Guided self-help is a useful first step, with education and support, often in a group setting.

## Prognosis

The prognosis is generally very good unless there are problems of low self-esteem or severe personality disorder.

## The SCOFF questionnaire[6]

These questions are useful as a screening tool for eating disorders, and can be used in any setting. A positive answer to two or more questions indicates that a further, more detailed history is indicated before considering treatment.

- Question 1.  Do you make yourself Sick because you feel uncomfortably full?
- Question 2.  Do you worry that you have lost Control over how much you eat?
- Question 3.  Have you recently lost more than One stone in a 3-month period?
- Question 4.  Do you believe yourself to be Fat when others say you are too thin?
- Question 5.  Would you say that Food dominates your life?

⊃ People with bulimia nervosa, p. 92.

## Reference

6  Morgan JF, Reid F and Lacey JH. The SCOFF questionnaire: assessment of a new screening tool for eating disorders. *British Medical Journal* 1999; **319**: 1467–8.

## Further reading

Duker M and Slade R. *Anorexia Nervosa and Bulimia*, 2nd edn. Open University Press: Buckingham, 2002.
Semple D and Smyth R (eds). *Oxford Handbook of Psychiatry*, 4th edn. Oxford University Press: Oxford, 2013.

# Schizophrenia

Schizophrenia is a highly variable disorder characterized by disordered perception, disordered thoughts (hallucinations and delusions), and withdrawal of the individual's interest from other people and the outside world.

Schizophrenia is a form of psychosis. Psychiatrists usually talk about 'schizophrenias', given the variability of this disorder. It typically develops in the late teens or early twenties, although males tend to have an earlier onset than females, and may develop more serious illness. Before the appearance of diagnosable symptoms, there is sometimes, particularly in young people, a period during which a prodrome of non-specific thoughts, behaviours, and feelings occur (such as loss of interest, avoiding the company of others, behaving irrationally or out of character, being irritable, and/or being over-sensitive). These symptoms are not diagnostic of any particular disorder, but they are not typical of the healthy state of the individual. They are often just as distressing to the family, and as incapacitating, as the delusions and hallucinations that develop later.

The symptoms of schizophrenia are divided into positive (active) symptoms and negative (loss of or withdrawal from previous function) symptoms (see Table 7.4).

**Table 7.4**  Symptoms of schizophrenia

| Positive symptoms | Negative symptoms | Other symptoms |
| --- | --- | --- |
| Delusions | Loss of motivation | Thought disorder |
| Hallucinations | Loss of social awareness | Agitation |
| | Loss of experience of pleasure | Depression |
| | | Poor sleep |
| | Flattened mood | Cognitive impairment |
| | Poor abstract thinking | Loss of libido |

The symptoms listed in Table 7.5 have a special significance for diagnosis, as they occur often in schizophrenia and more rarely in other disorders (they are sometimes referred to as first-rank symptoms).

The classification and diagnosis of schizophrenia was revised in 2013, so DSM-5 does not contain subtype classifications. Table 7.6 highlights the changes.

Table 7.5 First-rank symptoms of schizophrenia

| Key symptoms | |
| --- | --- |
| Auditory hallucinations | Voices heard arguing |
| | Thought echo |
| | Running commentary on what the person is doing |
| Delusions or thought interference | Thought insertion |
| | Thought withdrawal |
| | Thought broadcasting |
| Delusions of control | Passivity of affect |
| | Passivity of impulse |
| | Passivity of volitions |
| | Somatic passivity |
| Delusional perceptions | A primary delusion of any context reported by the person as having arisen from a normal perception |

## Epidemiology

- Prevalence—lifetime risk is 7–13 per 1000 members of the population.
- Mortality—suicide is the most common cause of premature death, accounting for 10–38% of all deaths.
- Genetic factors—account for 46% of identical twins, 40% both parents, 12–25% one parent, 12–15% sibling or non-identical twin, 6% grandparent, and 0.5–1% no relative affected.
- Environmental factors—complications of pregnancy, delivery, and the neonatal period, delayed walking and neurodevelopmental difficulties, early social services contact and disturbed childhood behaviour, and winter births.

## Prognosis

- Approximately 15–20% of first episodes will not recur.
- Few people with schizophrenia will remain in employment.
- Around 52% will not have experienced psychotic symptoms in the last 2 years.
- Around 52% are without negative symptoms.
- Around 55% show good or fair social functioning.

*Poor prognostic factors* include poor premorbid adjustment, insidious onset, early onset, cognitive impairment, and enlarged ventricles.

*Good prognostic factors* include marked mood disturbance (especially elation during initial presentation), family history of affective disorder, female gender, and living in a developed country.

➜ People with a perceptual disorder, p. 84.

Table 7.6 Revisions from DSM-IV to DSM-5

| ICD-10 | DSM-IV | DSM-5 | Key symptoms |
|---|---|---|---|
| Schizoaffective disorder | | All subtypes of schizophrenia deleted (paranoid, disorganized, catatonic, undifferentiated, and residual) | Abnormal thought processes and deregulated emotions—diagnosis is made when there are features of thought and mood disorders (either bipolar or depression) |
| Post-schizophrenia-depression | | | Residual positive and/or negative symptoms, but depression dominates |
| Catatonic schizophrenia | Catatonic type | No longer recognized as a separate disorder. It is associated with schizophrenia, bipolar disorder, PTSD, and depression, as well as with drug abuse or overdose, or abrupt or rapid withdrawal from benzodiazepines | Psychomotor disturbance, such as mutism, posturing, rigidity, staring, and stupor (apathetic state). Malignant—an acute onset of excitement, fear, autonomic instability, and delirium, and may be fatal |
| Paranoid schizophrenia | Paranoid type | Subtype deleted | Delusions and hallucinations |
| Hebephrenic schizophrenia | Disorganized type | Subtype deleted | Disorganized speech and behaviour (often silly or shallow), with flat or inappropriate manner |
| Undifferentiated schizophrenia | Undifferentiated type | Subtype deleted | |
| Residual schizophrenia | Residual type | Subtype deleted | Previous positive symptoms less marked, with prominent negative symptoms |
| Simple schizophrenia | | | No delusions or hallucinations; negative symptoms gradually arise without an acute episode |

## Further reading

Kingdon D and Turkington D. *Cognitive Therapy of Schizophrenia (Guides to Individualized Evidence-Based Treatment)*. The Guilford Press: New York, 2005.
Parker I et al. *Deconstructing Psychopathology*. London: Sage, 1995.

# Depression

In everyday language, 'depression' refers to any downturn in mood; it may be relatively transitory and perhaps due to something trivial. Clinical depression is different. It is marked by symptoms that last for 2 weeks or more and are so severe that they interfere with daily living. It is not secondary to the use of drugs or alcohol.

## Core symptoms of depression

- Depressed mood—present for most of the day, nearly every day, with little variation, and little responsiveness to environmental changes. There may be diurnal variation in mood (worse in the morning and improving as the day goes on).
- Anhedonia—diminished interest or pleasure in all, or almost all, activities for most of the day, nearly every day (based on subjective account or observation by others).
- Weight change—loss of weight when not dieting, or a weight gain (of more than 5% of body weight within a month) associated with an increase or decrease in appetite.
- Disturbed sleep—insomnia with early-morning wakening (2–3 hours earlier than usual) or hypersomnia, especially in atypical depression.
- Psychomotor agitation or retardation—observable by others, not just subjective feelings of restlessness or being slowed down.
- Fatigue or loss of energy.
- Feelings of worthlessness, or excessive inappropriate guilt (which may be delusional)—not just self-reproach or guilt about being ill.
- Reduced libido.
- Diminished ability to think or concentrate.
- Indecisiveness.
- Recurrent thoughts of death or suicide (not fear of dying), which may or may not have been acted upon.

Some of these symptoms are described as 'somatic' or biological, such as anhedonia, loss of emotional reactivity, early-morning wakening, and loss of appetite, weight, and libido.

## Psychotic symptoms

- Delusions—poverty, personal inadequacy, guilt, and assumed responsibility for world events, accidents, or natural disasters.
- Hallucinations—auditory (defamatory or accusatory voices), olfactory (bad smells such as rotting food or faeces), visual (tormentors, demons, dead bodies).
- Catatonic symptoms—marked psychomotor retardation (depressive stupor).

## Aetiology

Depression is likely to be caused by an interplay of biological, psychological, and social factors:

- *Genetic factors*—individual's sensitivity to life stressors.
- *Personality factors*—enduring traits with a biological basis, such as a positive attitude, or being 'laid back', which mediates the person's response to external stimuli or events.
- *Psychological factors*—the disruption of normal social, intimate, parental, or familial relationships is correlated with high rates of depression.
- *Gender*—there is an increased prevalence in women, possibly due to restricted social and occupational roles, ruminative response styles, and endocrine factors, or it may be that women are more likely to admit to these types of problems.
- *Social factors*—lower levels of income, employment, and education are predisposing factors; the stress associated with these problems leads to depression.
- *Social isolation*—a key risk factor, especially for those who already have an established mental health problem.

## Prognosis

Suicide rates vary, but are up to 13% for people with severe depression, and higher for individuals who have required hospital admission.

*Good prognostic factors*—acute onset, endogenous depression (from within, not related to an external event), and young age.

*Poor prognostic factors*—slow onset, neurotic features, elderly, residual symptoms, low confidence, alcohol or drug misuse, personality disorders, physical illness, or lack of social support.

➔ People with a mood disorder, p. 86.

## Further reading

National Institute for Mental Health. ℘ www.nimh.nih.gov
Semple D and Smyth R (eds). *Oxford Handbook of Psychiatry*, 4th edn. Oxford University Press: Oxford, 2013.

# Substance misuse

Substance misuse refers to the harmful use of any substance, such as alcohol or a street drug, or the misuse of a prescribed drug.

## Features of substance misuse disorder

- *Acute intoxication*—the pattern of reversible physical and mental abnormalities caused by the direct effect of the substance, such as disinhibition, ataxia, euphoria, and visual and sensory distortion.
- *At-risk use*—a pattern of substance use where the person is at increased risk of harming their physical or mental health. This can be normal consumption or harmful use. It does not depend on the amount taken, but on the situation and associated behaviours (e.g. alcohol and driving).
- *Harmful use*—the continuation of substance misuse despite evidence of damage to the person's mental health or their social, occupational, or familial well-being. Damage is denied or minimized.
- *Dependence*—includes both physical and psychological dependence.
- *Withdrawal*—physical dependence where abstinence leads to features of withdrawal. Different substances produce different withdrawal symptoms, which are often the opposite of the acute effects of the substance. Clinically significant withdrawal is associated with abstinence from alcohol, opiates, benzodiazepines, amphetamines, and cocaine.
- *Complicated withdrawal*—development of seizures, delirium, or psychotic features.
- *Substance-induced psychotic disorder*—hallucinations and/or delusions occurring as a direct result of substance neurotoxicity. Features may occur during intoxication or withdrawal states. It is differentiated from primary psychotic illness by the symptoms being non-typical (e.g. late first presentation, prominence of non-auditory hallucinations).
- *Cognitive impairment syndromes*—reversible cognitive deficits that occur during intoxication, and that persist in chronic misuse, resulting in a dementia syndrome. They are most commonly associated with misuse of alcohol, volatile chemicals, benzodiazepines, and possibly cannabis.
- *Residual disorders*—symptoms that persist despite discontinuation of the substance.
- *Exacerbation of pre-existing disorder*—all other psychiatric illnesses, especially anxiety, panic disorders, mood disorders, and psychotic disorders, may be associated with comorbid substance misuse. This results in exacerbation of the patient's symptoms and a decline in the effectiveness of treatment.

### Dependence syndrome

Dependence syndrome is a collective term for the following features of substance dependence:

- Primacy of drug-seeking behaviour—the drug is the most important thing in the person's life, taking priority over all activities and interests.
- Narrowing the drug-taking repertoire—the person takes a single substance in preference to all others.

- Increased tolerance to the effects of the drug—increased amounts are needed to achieve the same effect, and the person explores other routes of administration, such as intravenous injection.
- Loss of control of consumption—there is an inability to restrict further consumption.
- Signs of withdrawal when the person attempts to abstain from the drug.
- Drug taking to avoid withdrawal symptoms.
- Continued drug use despite negative consequences, such as relationship breakdown, prison sentence, or loss of job.
- Rapid reinstatement of the previous pattern of drug use after abstinence.

➔ People with substance misuse problems, p. 94.

## Further reading

Chick J. *Understanding Alcohol and Drinking Problems*. British Medical Association: London, 2006.
Semple D and Smyth R (eds). *Oxford Handbook of Psychiatry*, 4th edn. Oxford University Press: Oxford, 2013.

# Personality disorder

The term 'personality disorder' (PD) is contentious, and in the past the term has been used as a pejorative label for 'patients who are unpopular'. DSM-5 now defines personality disorders as enduring patterns of behaviours, cognitions, and inner experiences that are severely out of context and deviate from those accepted by an individual's culture.[7]

Diagnostic reliability remains poor. To support clearer diagnostic criteria and stimulate further research, Section 3 of DSM-5 outlines a hybrid dimensional–categorical PD model.[7]

PDs begin in childhood or adolescence and continue into adulthood. They are persistent pervasive disorders of inner experience and behaviour that cause distress or significant impairment of social functioning.

A PD can be manifested by problems in the following areas:

• Cognition—ways of perceiving and thinking about oneself and others.
• Affect—the range, intensity, and appropriateness of emotional response.
• Behaviour—interpersonal, occupational, and social functioning.

As there are many definition categories, there are problems with regard to classifying PDs. There are also conflicting views[8] about their diagnosis (see Tables 7.7 and 7.8). Nevertheless, despite the controversy, the National Institute for Health and Care Excellence (NICE) now stipulates that people with borderline personality disorder should not be excluded from any health or social care service because of their diagnosis or because they have self-harmed.[9]

**Table 7.7** Arguments for and against the diagnosis of personality disorder

| Arguments for the diagnosis | Arguments against the diagnosis |
| --- | --- |
| People with PD suffer with the symptoms of their condition | Personality is by definition unchangeable |
| There is a high rate of suicide, premature death, and other mental illness associated with PD | There is no evidence that psychiatric treatment can have any impact on PD |
| Some treatment approaches are effective | People with PD are disruptive and have a negative impact on staff and other patients |
| Traditional services do not provide the type of approach that is required | People with PD are not ill, and are therefore responsible for their behaviour |
|  | PDs are basically a social problem |

**Table 7.8** Classification of personality disorder

| Personality disorder | Description |
|---|---|
| Paranoid | Sensitive, suspicious, preoccupied with conspiratorial explanations, self-referential, distrusting of others |
| Schizoid | Emotionally cold, detached, lack of interest in others, excessive introspection and fantasy |
| Schizotypal | Interpersonal discomfort with peculiar ideas, perceptions, appearance, and behaviours |
| Antisocial | Callous lack of concern for others, irresponsibility, irritability, aggression, inability to maintain enduring relationships, disregard and violation of others' rights, evidence of childhood conduct disorder |
| Emotionally unstable | Inability to control anger or pain, with unpredictable affect and behaviour |
| Borderline | Unclear identity, intense and unstable relationships, unpredictable affect, frequent threats and acts of self-harm, impulsivity |
| Histrionic | Self-dramatization, shallow affect, egocentricity, craving attention and excitement, manipulative behaviour |
| Narcissistic | Grandiosity, lack of empathy, need for admiration |
| Avoidant | Tension, self-consciousness, fear of negative evaluation by others, timidity and insecurity |
| Obsessive–compulsive | Doubt, indecisiveness, caution, pedantry, rigidity, perfectionism, preoccupation with orderliness and control |
| Dependent | Clinging, submissive, excessive need for care, feeling of helplessness when not in a relationship |

## Aetiology

There is no single theory for the causes of PD. However, the following factors may be relevant:

- Genetics—there is some evidence of a link between affective disorder and borderline personality disorder, and between delusional disorder and paranoid personality disorder.
- Childhood development—a difficult temperament in infancy may proceed to conduct disorder in childhood and personality disorder in adulthood. Attention deficit hyperactivity disorder (ADHD) and family pathology are possible risk factors for antisocial personality disorder, and sexual abuse may increase the risk of developing borderline personality disorder.
- Psychodynamic theories—these are Freudian explanations of arrested development at the oral, anal, and genital stages leading to narcissistic and borderline personality with primitive defence mechanisms and projective identification (including splitting).

- Cognitive behaviour theories—maladaptive core beliefs are derived from an interaction between childhood experience and pre-programmed patterns of behaviour.
- Cognitive analytical model—people experience a range of partially dissociated self states in response to unmanageable external threats.
- Dialectical behaviour model—innate temperamental vulnerabilities interact with dysfunctional invalidating environments, resulting in problems with emotional regulation.

➔ People with personality disorder, p. 98.

## References

7   American Psychiatric Association. *Highlights of Changes from DSM-IV-TR to DSM-5*. American Psychiatric Publishing: Arlington, VA, 2012. ℅ www.dsm5.org/Documents/changes%20from%20dsm-iv-tr%20to%20dsm-5.pdf

8   Schacter DL, Gilbert DT and Wegner DM. *Psychology*, 2nd edn. Worth Publishers: New York, 2011.

9   National Institute for Health and Care Excellence (NICE). *Borderline Personality Disorder: treatment and management*. CG78. NICE: London, 2009. ℅ www.nice.org.uk/Guidance/CG78

## Further reading

Lieb K et al. Pharmacotherapy for borderline personality disorder: Cochrane systematic review of randomised trials. *British Journal of Psychiatry* 2010; **196**: 4–12.

Sharpe R. *A Fractured Mind: my life with multiple personality disorder*. Souvenir Press Ltd: London, 2006.

Stoffers JM et al. Psychological therapies for people with borderline personality disorder. *Cochrane Database of Systematic Reviews* 2012; **8**: CD005652.

# Bipolar disorder

People with bipolar disorder can experience recurrent episodes of depression and mania or hypomania. The disorder used to be called manic depression, and is more common in women, with an average age of onset of around 21 years. Children of a parent with bipolar disorder have a 50% probability of developing a mental illness. There are no significant differences between racial groups.

The course of the illness is extremely variable. The onset can be hypomanic, manic, mixed, or depressive, and this may be followed by a period of 5 or more years without a further episode. The time interval between episodes may then begin to decrease. People with hypomania have the same symptoms as those with mania, but to a lesser degree, and the condition may not significantly disrupt work or lead to social rejection.

## Core features of mania

- Elevated mood, usually out of keeping with circumstances.
- Increased energy, which may manifest as:
  - overactivity
  - pressured speech (flight of ideas)
  - racing thoughts
  - reduced need for sleep.
- Increased self-esteem, which manifests as:
  - overoptimistic ideation
  - grandiosity
  - reduced social inhibition
  - overfamiliarity (may be over-amorous)
  - facetiousness.
- Reduced attention span or increased distractibility.
- Tendency to engage in high-risk behaviour that could have serious consequences, such as:
  - preoccupation with extravagant impractical schemes
  - spending recklessly
  - inappropriate sexual encounters.
- Other behavioural manifestations:
  - excitement
  - irritability
  - aggressiveness or suspiciousness.
- Disruption of work, usual social activities, and family life.

## Psychotic symptoms

In severe mania, psychotic symptoms may develop.

- Grandiose ideas may become delusional, with special powers or religious content.
- Suspiciousness may develop into well-formed persecutory delusions.
- Pressured speech may become so great that clear associations are lost and speech becomes incomprehensible.
- Irritability and aggression may lead to violent behaviour.
- Preoccupation with thoughts and schemes may lead to self-neglect to the point of not eating or drinking, and living in dishevelled circumstances.
- Catatonic behaviour, also termed manic stupor, may occur.
- There is total loss of insight and connection to the outside world.

## Prognosis

Morbidity rates are high in terms of lost work, productivity, and effects on relationships and the family. Mortality rates are also high. Around 25–50% of people with bipolar disorder attempt suicide, and 10% die as a result of suicide.

*Poor prognostic factors* include poor employment history, alcohol abuse, psychotic features, depression between episodes of mania, being male, and not complying with medication.

*Good prognostic factors* include manic episodes of short duration, later age of onset, few thoughts of suicide or symptoms of psychosis, good treatment response, and compliance.

## Further reading

Fink C and Kraynak J. *Bipolar Disorder for Dummies*, 2nd edn. John Wiley & Sons Ltd: New York, 2012.
Miklowitz DJ. *The Bipolar Disorder Survival Guide: what you and your family need to know*, 2nd edn. The Guilford Press: New York, 2011.
Semple D and Smyth R (eds). *Oxford Handbook of Psychiatry*, 4th edn. Oxford University Press: Oxford, 2013.

# Obsessive–compulsive disorder

### Definition

The essential feature of this disorder is recurrent obsessional thoughts or compulsive acts. Obsessional thoughts are ideas, images, or impulses that enter a person's mind again and again. They are distressing because they are intrusive and irrational, and they may be violent or obscene. People can usually recognize their thoughts and compulsions as unreasonable and excessive, and often try unsuccessfully to resist them.

The average age of onset of obsessive–compulsive disorder (OCD) is around 20 years. The prevalence of the disorder in the population is 0.5–2%, with an equal male:female distribution. The course of the condition is variable, and is more likely to be chronic in the absence of significant depressive symptoms.

### Core features of OCD

- The obsessions or compulsions must be recognized as the person's own thoughts or impulses, even though they may be involuntary or repugnant.
- There must be at least one thought or act that is still resisted successfully, even though others may be present which the person no longer resists.
- Carrying out the compulsive act must not in itself be pleasurable (simple relief of tension or anxiety is not regarded as pleasure in this sense).
- The thoughts, images, or impulses must be intrusive and unpleasantly repetitive.

### Categories or types of OCD

- Checking.
- Washing.
- Contamination.
- Doubting.
- Body dysmorphic (including repetitive behaviours or mental acts that may arise with regard to perceived defects or flaws in the person's physical appearance).
- Counting.
- Insistence on symmetry.
- Aggressive thoughts.
- Hoarding.
- Excoriation (skin picking).
- Trichotillomania (hair-pulling disorder).

### Compulsions

Compulsive acts or rituals are stereotyped behaviours that are repeated again and again. They are not inherently enjoyable, nor do they result in the completion of an inherently useful task. Repeated attempts are made to resist the behaviour. However, in very long-standing cases, resistance may be minimal. Autonomic anxiety symptoms are often present, but distressing feelings of internal or psychic tension without obvious autonomic arousal are also common.

## Depression

There is a close relationship between compulsions and obsessional symptoms, particularly obsessional thoughts, and depression. People with OCD often have depressive symptoms, and those who have recurrent depressive disorder may develop obsessional thoughts during their episodes of depression. In either situation, increases or decreases in the severity of the depressive symptoms are generally accompanied by parallel changes in the severity of the obsessional symptoms.

## Prognosis

- Around 20–40% of cases improve significantly, and around 40–50% show a moderate improvement.
- Around 20–40% have chronic or worsening symptoms.
- Relapse rates are high if medication is stopped.

*Poor prognostic factors* include giving in to compulsions, longer duration, early onset, bizarre compulsions, symmetry, comorbid depression, and personality disorder.

*Better prognostic factors* include good premorbid social and occupational adjustment, a precipitating event, and episodic symptoms.

## Further reading

Deane R. *Washing My Life Away: surviving obsessive–compulsive disorder.* Jessica Kingsley Publishers: London, 2005.
Semple D and Smyth R (eds). *Oxford Handbook of Psychiatry*, 4th edn. Oxford University Press: Oxford, 2013.
Zohar J (ed.). *Obsessive Compulsive Disorder: current science and clinical practice.* John Wiley & Sons Ltd: Chichester, 2012.

# Anxiety

## Definition

Anxiety is a normal and adaptive response to stress and danger. It is damaging if it is prolonged, severe, or out of proportion to the real threat of the external situation. Moderate amounts of anxiety can optimize performance (e.g. being nervous before a test or exam may help you to perform better). The sensations of anxiety are related to autonomic arousal and cognitive appraisal of threat, which were adaptive primitive survival mechanisms. This is referred to as the 'fight or flight' instinct.

Anxiety has two components:
- Psychic anxiety—subjective tension, increased arousal, and fearful apprehension.
- Somatic anxiety—bodily sensations such as palpitations, sweating, dyspnoea (shortness of breath), pallor, or abdominal discomfort.

## Symptoms of anxiety

*General symptoms of anxiety and tension*—hot flushes or cold chills, numbness or tingling sensations, muscle tension, aches and pains, restlessness or an inability to relax, feeling keyed up, on edge, or mentally tense, a sensation of a lump in the throat, or difficulty swallowing.

*Physical symptoms*—breathing difficulties, dry mouth, palpitations, choking sensation, chest pain or discomfort, tachycardia, sweating, trembling, nausea, and abdominal distress.

*Mental state symptoms*—feeling dizzy, unsteady, faint, or light-headed, fear of losing control, 'going crazy', passing out, or dying.

*Other symptoms*—exaggerated response to minor surprises or being startled, concentration difficulties, mind going blank due to worry or anxiety, persistent irritability, and difficulty getting to sleep due to worry.

## Anxiety disorders

### Generalized anxiety disorder (GAD)

This is characterized by excessive worry (free-floating and persistent), feelings of apprehension about everyday events or problems, and symptoms of muscle and psychic tension, causing significant distress and functional impairment.

### Acute stress reaction

This is a transient disorder that may last for hours or days, and that may occur as an immediate response (within 1 hour) to exceptional circumstances (e.g. after a major accident, assault, warfare, or rape). The stressor usually involves a severe threat to the security or physical integrity of the individual or a loved one.

### Acute stress disorder

This overlaps with acute stress reaction, with an emphasis on the symptoms of dissociation and hyperarousal. Onset is usually within 4 weeks of an event, with symptoms lasting for up to 4 weeks, after which post-traumatic stress disorder (PTSD) has to be considered.

*Panic attack*

This is characterized by a period of intense fear, which develops rapidly and reaches a peak of intensity at around 10 minutes (it does not generally last longer than 20–30 minutes). A panic attack may be spontaneous or situational, and can occur during sleep.

*Panic disorder*

This is diagnosed when a person has recurrent panic attacks that are not secondary to substance misuse, a medical condition, or another mental health problem.

➲ People with anxiety disorders, p. 88.

## Further reading

Marks I. *Living with Fear: understanding and coping with anxiety*, 2nd edn. McGraw-Hill Publishing Company: Maidenhead, 2005.

Semple D and Smyth R (eds). *Oxford Handbook of Psychiatry*, 4th edn. Oxford University Press: Oxford, 2013.

# Phobias

## Definition

Phobias are caused by fear of particular stimuli, events, or situations. The fear arouses symptoms of anxiety, and the situations or stimuli are therefore associated with avoidance. The concept of biological preparedness is that some fears (e.g. of snakes, fire, and heights) had an evolutionary advantage.

## Signs

- Somatic physical symptoms, such as blushing, trembling, or dry mouth, when exposed to the object or situation. Anxiety reactions (e.g. sweating, trembling, nausea, rapid heartbeat) are common.
- Excessive fear (that is recognized as excessive by the individual) of humiliation, embarrassment, or others noticing how anxious they are.
- Affected individuals characteristically have a critical and perfectionist personality.
- Difficulty in maintaining social or sexual relationships, educational problems, difficulties in interactions with others, or problems at work, caused by avoidance.
- Thoughts of suicide are relatively common.

## Specific phobias

People with specific phobias experience excessive and unreasonable psychological or autonomic symptoms of severe anxiety and panic in the presence or anticipated presence of a specific feared object or situation, which leads to avoidance.

Phobias may begin in childhood, and are often brought on by a traumatic event (e.g. being bitten by a dog may bring about a fear of dogs). Phobias that begin in childhood may disappear as the person grows older. There are four common categories of phobia:

- Fear of animals—for example, fear of human hair (trichophobia), animal fur (chaetophobia), or skin (doraphobia).
- Fear of aspects of the natural environment—for example, fear of the dark (nyctophobia).
- Fear of blood, injury, or injection (trypanophobia).
- Fear of specific situations—for example, the dentist (dentophobia) or hospitals (nosocomephobia).

Other common phobias include fear of choking (anginophobia) and deep water (bathophobia).

## Social phobia

Social phobia is experienced as symptoms of incapacitating anxiety, which are not secondary to delusional or obsessive thoughts. These are restricted to particular social situations, leading to a desire for escape or avoidance (which may reinforce a strongly held belief of social inadequacy). The onset of this phobia is usually in mid to late adolescence.

## Agoraphobia

Agoraphobia sometimes coexists with panic disorder. It is characterized by a fear of having a panic attack in a place from which it is difficult to escape. Many people with agoraphobia refuse to leave their home, often for years at a time. Others develop a fixed route, or territory, from which they cannot deviate, such as the route between home and work. It becomes impossible to travel beyond what they consider to be their safety zone without experiencing severe anxiety.

## Claustrophobia

One of the most common phobias is claustrophobia—a fear of enclosed spaces. A person who has claustrophobia may panic when inside a lift, an aeroplane, a crowded room, or another confined area. For a person with severe claustrophobia, a closed door may trigger feelings of panic.

*Common claustrophobic behaviour*
- *Inside a room*—automatically checking for the exits, standing near the exits, or feeling alarmed when all of the doors are closed.
- *Inside a vehicle*—avoiding public transport or times when traffic is known to be heavy.
- *Inside a building*—preferring to take the stairs rather than the lift.
- *At a party*—standing near the door in a crowded room, even if the room is large and spacious.

## Further reading

Beck A and Emery G. *Anxiety Disorders and Phobias: a cognitive perspective*, 15th anniversary edn. Basic Books: New York, 2005.

# Sexual disorders: female

The primary characteristic of female sexual disorder is impairment of normal sexual functioning. This can refer to an inability to reach orgasm, painful sexual intercourse, strong feelings of repulsion with regard to sexual activity, or an exaggerated sexual response cycle or sexual interest. For a diagnosis of sexual dysfunction to be made, the symptoms must be hindering the person's everyday functioning, and any possible medical cause must be ruled out.

## Female orgasmic disorder

*Aetiology*

In women, inability to reach orgasm is related to intimacy issues, feelings of fear and anxiety, and a sense of not being safe within the intimate relationship or within relationships in general.

*Symptoms*

There is a delay in orgasm following normal excitement and sexual activity. Due to the wide variation in sexual response in women, it must be judged by a clinician to be significant, taking into account the person's age and situation. For this diagnosis to be made, the condition must be persistent or occur frequently and cause significant distress. Substance abuse must be ruled out.

*Treatment*

Typical treatment involves discovering and resolving underlying conflicts or life difficulties through counselling or psychotherapy.

*Prognosis*

The prognosis is very good, especially if the underlying issues are addressed and worked through.

## Female sexual arousal disorder

*Aetiology*

There is some evidence to suggest that relationship problems and/or sexual trauma in childhood may play a role in the development of this disorder.

*Symptoms*

Until sexual activity is complete, there is an inability to attain or maintain adequate lubrication in response to sexual excitement. For this diagnosis to be made, the condition must result in significant distress and not be better accounted for by another disorder (e.g. oestrogen depletion) or the misuse of a substance.

*Treatment*

Typical treatment involves discovering and resolving underlying conflict or life difficulties (e.g. with the help of a therapist).

*Prognosis*

This varies, but it improves with the ability to gain insight into and work through relationship problems or problems stemming from childhood which are playing a role in the disorder.

## Vaginismus

### Aetiology
There is a relationship between this disorder and having been the victim of rape or sexual abuse, a history of strict religious upbringing, and issues of control.

### Symptoms
Recurrent or persistent involuntary spasms of the vaginal muscles interfere with sexual intercourse. For this diagnosis to be made, the condition must be causing significant distress, and other medical conditions or disorders must be ruled out.

### Treatment
Psychological treatment involves working through the underlying issues. Other treatments can involve the use of progressively larger dilators, and therapy to help to relax the muscles which are preventing intercourse.

### Prognosis
The prognosis is good.

➲ Assessing and managing the side effects of medication, p. 264.
➲ Sexuality and mental health: a research study, p. 276.
➲ Sexuality (sexual orientation) and mental health, p. 278.

## Further reading
AllPsych Online. ℘ www.allpsych.com
ICON Health Publications. *Female Sexual Dysfunction: a medical dictionary, bibliography and annotated research guide to Internet references.* ICON Health Publications: San Diego, CA, 2004.

# Sexual disorders: male

## Male orgasmic disorder

### Aetiology

Male orgasmic disorder is often thought of as beginning in adolescence or early adulthood, especially if sexual intimacy becomes linked to a negative life event or aspect. A medical cause must always be ruled out first.

### Symptoms

There is delay or absence of orgasm following normal excitement and sexual activity. Due to the wide variation in sexual response in men, the symptom must be judged by a clinician to be significant, taking into account the person's age and situation. For a diagnosis to be made, the condition must be persistent or occur frequently and cause significant distress. The effect of substance abuse must also be ruled out.

### Treatment

Once a medical cause has been ruled out, working through the underlying issues can be very helpful. If the underlying issues are not significant, some therapists also use behavioural techniques such as sensate focus, which is a more direct approach.

### Prognosis

The prognosis is very good.

## Male erectile disorder (impotence)

### Aetiology

Any medical causes of this disorder (which was previously known as impotence) must be ruled out first. In the absence of any physiological cause, male erectile disorder is typically a result of 'performance anxiety' or fear of not being able to achieve or maintain an erection.

### Symptoms

There is a recurring inability to achieve or maintain an erection until sexual activity is complete. For a diagnosis to be made, the condition must be causing significant distress for the individual, and other disorders such as drug abuse or a physical problem must be ruled out.

### Treatment

The most commonly used treatment for non-medical-related male erectile disorder is the 'sensate focus' technique, taught by a qualified sex therapist or counsellor. This involves a gradual progression of sexual intimacy, typically over the course of several weeks, eventually leading to penetration and orgasm.

### Prognosis

The prognosis is very good.

## Premature ejaculation

### Aetiology

Any medical causes must be ruled out first. Relationship stress, a new relationship, anxiety, and issues related to control and intimacy can all play a role in the development of this disorder.

### Symptoms

Ejaculation occurs with minimal sexual stimulation, before or shortly after penetration and before the person wishes it to occur. For this diagnosis to be made the condition must be persistent or occur frequently and cause significant distress. The effect of substance use must also be ruled out.

### Treatment

The treatment options include relaxation training, education, and working through the underlying issues. If the relationship is new, the difficulties will often resolve as the relationship matures.

### Prognosis

The prognosis is good.

⬇ Assessing and managing the side effects of medication, p. 264.
⬇ Sexuality and mental health: a research study, p. 276.
⬇ Sexuality (sexual orientation) and mental health, p. 278.

## Further reading

AllPsych Online. ♪ www.allpsych.com
ICON Health Publications. *Male Sexual Dysfunction: a medical dictionary, bibliography and annotated research guide to Internet references.* ICON Health Publications: San Diego, CA, 2004.

# Sexual disorders: female and male

## Gender identity disorder

### Aetiology

A number of theories suggest that childhood issues may play a role in this disorder—for example, the early parent–child relationship, and the child's identification with the parent of the same gender.

### Symptoms

There is a strong and persistent identification with the opposite gender. The person feels a sense of discomfort in their own gender, and may feel that they were 'born the wrong sex'. This disorder has been confused with cross-dressing or transvestic fetishism, but these are all separate conditions. Depression, anxiety, relationship difficulties, and personality disorders may also coexist with gender identity disorder. Homosexuality is present in the majority of cases.

### Treatment

Psychological treatment is likely to be long term, with small gains made on underlying issues as treatment progresses. Gender reassignment is suitable for a minority of sufferers.

### Prognosis

The prognosis is mixed. The goals of treatment are not as clear as in other disorders, as same-sex identification may be very difficult to achieve. More achievable goals may include an acceptance of the assigned gender, and resolution of other difficulties such as depression or anxiety.

## Hypoactive sexual desire disorder

### Aetiology

Some evidence suggests that relationship issues and/or sexual trauma in childhood may play a role in the development of this disorder. Life stressors or other interpersonal difficulties may also contribute.

### Symptoms

The diagnosis must be made by a clinician, taking into account the individual's age and life circumstances. The lack of desire experienced must result in significant distress for the individual, and another disorder or physical problem must be ruled out.

### Treatment

Typical treatment would involve discovering and resolving any underlying conflict or life difficulties *through counselling or therapy*.

### Prognosis

The course of this disorder can be consistent or periodic, and it can therefore resurface after a period of remission if relationship problems or life stressors re-emerge.

## Sexual aversion disorder

*Aetiology*

Some evidence suggests that relationship problems and/or sexual trauma in childhood may play a role in the development of this disorder.

*Symptoms*

There is a persistent or recurring aversion to, or avoidance of, sexual activity. When presented with a sexual opportunity, the person may experience panic attacks or extreme anxiety. This aversion must result in significant distress for the individual, and other disorders and physical problems must be ruled out.

*Treatment*

Typical treatment would involve discovering and resolving the underlying conflict or life difficulties *through counselling or therapy*.

*Prognosis*

The prognosis improves with the ability to gain insight and work through relationship problems, or issues stemming from childhood, which are playing a role in this disorder.

➔ Assessing and managing the side effects of medication, p. 264.

➔ Sexuality and mental health: a research study, p. 276.

➔ Sexuality (sexual orientation) and mental health, p. 278.

## Further reading

Dickinson T, Cook M, Playle J and Hallett C. 'Queer' treatments: giving a voice to former patients who received treatments for their 'sexual deviations'. *Journal of Clinical Nursing* 2012; **21**: 1345–54.

Plaut M, Graziottin A and Heaton PW. *Fast Facts: sexual dysfunction.* Health Press Ltd: Oxford, 2004.

# Somatoform disorders

Somatoform disorders are a group of disorders characterized by physical symptoms that suggest a medical condition. They are classified as psychiatric conditions because the physical symptoms present cannot be fully explained by a medical disorder, substance misuse, or another mental disorder.

## Body dysmorphic disorder

- There is a preoccupation with an imagined defect in the person's appearance. If a slight physical anomaly is present, the person is excessively concerned about it.
- This preoccupation with appearance causes clinically significant distress, or impairment in social, occupational, or other important areas of functioning.
- The preoccupation is not caused by another disorder (e.g. dissatisfaction with body shape and size in anorexia nervosa).

## Conversion disorder

- One or more symptoms or deficits affecting voluntary motor or sensory function are present, which suggest a neurological or other general medical condition.
- Psychological factors are judged to be associated with the symptom or deficit, because its appearance is preceded by conflicts or other stressors.
- The symptom or deficit is not intentionally produced or feigned (as in factitious disorder or malingering).
- The symptom or deficit cannot be fully explained (after appropriate investigation) by a general medical condition, as a culturally sanctioned behaviour or experience, or by the direct effects of substance misuse.
- The symptom or deficit causes clinically significant distress or impairment in social, occupational, or other important areas of functioning, or warrants medical intervention.
- The symptom or deficit is not limited to pain or sexual dysfunction, it does not occur exclusively during the course of somatization disorder (see later in this section), and it cannot be accounted for by another mental disorder.

## Hypochondriasis

- This is a preoccupation with the fear of having, or the idea that one has, a serious disease, based on a misinterpretation of bodily symptoms.
- The preoccupation persists despite appropriate medical evaluation and reassurance.
- The preoccupation causes clinically significant distress or impairment in social, occupational, or other important areas of functioning.
- The duration of the disturbance is at least 6 months.
- The preoccupation is not better accounted for by generalized anxiety disorder.

### Somatization disorder

There is a history of many physical complaints—beginning before the age of 30 years—that occur over a period of several years and result in treatment being sought, or in significant impairment in social, occupational, or other important areas of functioning.

Each of the following criteria must be met, with individual symptoms occurring at any time during the course of the disturbance:

• *Four pain symptoms*—a history of pain related to at least four different sites or functions (e.g. head, abdomen, back, joints, extremities, chest, rectum, during menstruation, during sexual intercourse, or during urination).

• *Two gastrointestinal symptoms*—a history of at least two gastrointestinal symptoms other than pain (e.g. nausea, bloating, vomiting other than during pregnancy, diarrhoea, or intolerance of several different foods).

• *One sexual symptom*—a history of at least one sexual or reproductive symptom other than pain (e.g. sexual indifference, erectile or ejaculatory dysfunction, irregular menses, excessive menstrual bleeding, vomiting throughout pregnancy).

• *One pseudoneurological symptom*—a history of at least one symptom or deficit suggesting a neurological condition, not limited to pain (e.g. conversion symptoms such as impaired coordination or balance, paralysis or localized weakness, difficulty swallowing, or loss of consciousness other than fainting).

➔ Working with specific physical and psychosomatic disorders, p. 396.

### Further reading

BehaveNet. ♫ www.behavenet.com

Lamberty GJ. *Understanding Somatization in the Practice of Clinical Neuropsychology.* AACN Workshop Series. Oxford University Press: Oxford, 2008.

# Neuropsychiatric disorders

Neuropsychiatry is at the interface of psychiatry and neurology. It is a specialist medical discipline that deals with the behavioural or psychological difficulties associated with known or suspected neurological conditions. Technically, neuropsychiatry focuses on abnormalities in the areas of higher brain function, such as the cerebral cortex and the limbic system.

## Epilepsy

Epilepsy (often referred to as a seizure disorder) is a chronic neurological condition characterized by recurrent unprovoked seizures. It is commonly controlled with medication, although surgical methods are also used.

Seizures can be sub-classified into a number of categories, depending on their behavioural effects

### Absence seizures

These are sometimes called 'petit mal' seizures. They involve an interruption to consciousness, where the person affected seems to become vacant and unresponsive for a short period of time (usually up to 30 seconds). Slight muscle twitching may occur.

### Tonic–clonic seizures

These are sometimes called 'grand mal' seizures. They involve an initial contraction of the muscles (the 'tonic' phase), which may result in tongue biting, urinary incontinence, and the absence of breathing. This is followed by rhythmic muscle contractions (the 'clonic' phase). The colloquial term 'epileptic fit' refers to this type of seizure.

### Myoclonic seizures

These involve sporadic muscle contraction and can result in jerky movements of muscles or muscle groups.

### Atonic seizures

These involve the loss of muscle tone, causing the person to fall to the ground. They are sometimes called 'drop attacks', but must be distinguished from similar looking attacks that may occur in narcolepsy or cataplexy.

### Status epilepticus

This refers to continuous seizure activity with no recovery between successive tonic–clonic seizures. This is a life-threatening condition, and if it is suspected, emergency medical assistance should be summoned immediately. A tonic–clonic seizure that lasts for longer than 5 minutes (or 2 minutes longer than the person's normal seizures) is usually considered grounds for calling the emergency services.

## Attention deficit hyperactivity disorder (ADHD)

ADHD is one of the most commonly diagnosed mental disorders in children. It may be diagnosed in adults if symptoms were present (even if undiagnosed) in childhood. Current theory holds that approximately 30% of children who are diagnosed with ADHD will retain the disorder as adults. In adulthood the condition is often referred to as adult attention deficit disorder (AADD).

## Tourette's syndrome

Tourette's syndrome is a neurological or neurochemical disorder character-ized by tics. These may be involuntary, rapid, sudden movements or vocali-zations that occur repeatedly in the same way. The onset is usually before the age of 18 years.

The tics can be almost any short vocal sound, but the most common ones resemble throat clearing, short coughs, grunts, or moans. Motor tics can be of endless variety and may include hand-clapping, banging the knuckles together, or contorted facial grimacing.

Vocal tics fall into a number of categories:

- *Echolalia*—the urge to repeat words spoken by someone else after they have been heard by the person with the disorder.
- *Palilalia*—the urge to repeat one's own previously spoken words.
- *Lexilalia*—the urge to repeat words after reading them.
- *Coprolalia*—the spontaneous utterance of socially offensive words, such as obscenities and racial or ethnic slurs.

Features of Tourette's syndrome include:

- Multiple motor tics and one or more vocal tics presenting at some time during the disorder, although not necessarily simultaneously.
- Tics occurring many times a day (usually in bouts), nearly every day or intermittently over a period of more than 1 year.
- Periodic changes in the number, frequency, type, and location of tics, and in the waxing and waning of their severity. Symptoms may disappear for weeks or months at a time.

## Tardive dyskinesia

Tardive dyskinesia is a serious neurological disorder caused by the long-term use of traditional antipsychotic (neuroleptic) drugs. The new generation of atypical antipsychotics appear to cause tardive dyskinesia less frequently.

Tardive dyskinesia is characterized by repetitive, involuntary, purposeless movements. Features of the disorder may include grimacing, tongue protru-sion, lip smacking, puckering and pursing of the lips, and rapid eye blinking. Rapid movements of the arms, legs, and trunk may also occur.

→ Assessment of children and adolescents, p. 146.
→ Interventions in child and adolescent mental health, p. 148.

## Further reading

Mitchell AJ. *Neuropsychiatry and Behavioral Neurology Explained*. Elsevier Health Sciences: Philadelphia, PA, 2003.

# Sleep disorders

A sleep disorder, also called somnipathy, is an interruption or disturbance in a person's usual sleep patterns. Some sleep disorders can interfere with mental and emotional functioning because they interfere with rapid eye movement (REM) sleep (see later in topic).

## Normal sleep stages

*Stage 1*

This is experienced as falling asleep, and is a transition stage between being awake and sleep. It lasts between 1 and 5 minutes and accounts for approximately 2–5% of a normal night of sleep.

*Stage 2*

This follows Stage 1 and is the 'baseline' of sleep. It is part of the 90-minute cycle (see later in topic) and accounts for approximately 45–60% of sleep.

*Stages 3 and 4*

Stage 2 sleep evolves into 'delta' sleep after approximately 10–20 minutes, and may last for 15–30 minutes. It is also called 'slow-wave' sleep, because brain activity slows down dramatically. In most adults, these two stages are completed within the first two 90-minute sleep cycles, or within the first 3 hours of sleep. Delta sleep is the 'deepest' and most restorative stage of sleep.

*Stage 5*

REM sleep is a very active stage of sleep and accounts for 20–25% of a normal night's sleep. Breathing, heart rate, and brainwave activity become faster, and vivid dreams can occur.

## Sleep cycles

A typical night's sleep includes four or five cycles of these sequential stages, each lasting between 90 and 110 minutes. As the night progresses, the amount of time spent in delta sleep decreases, with a corresponding increase in REM sleep.

## Insomnia

Insomnia is difficulty in going to sleep and/or maintaining sleep. The term 'insomnia' is often used to indicate all stages and types of sleep loss. Insomnia is a symptom, not a disorder.

*Primary insomnia*

Aetiology

Primary insomnia occurs in up to 10% of adults and in up to 25% of elderly adults. It appears to be slightly more common in women. There may be a different cause of primary insomnia for each individual, but it often involves a preoccupation with the inability to sleep, or excessive worry about sleep, which can cause the person to stay awake. Many people report that they sleep better away from home, which suggests that conditioning related to the bedroom has occurred. This can result in bouts of sleep while watching TV, being a passenger in a car, or in other areas not associated with the bedroom.

*Symptoms*

The criteria for a diagnosis of primary insomnia include difficulty falling asleep, remaining asleep, or experiencing restorative sleep for no less than 1 month. This disturbance in sleep must cause significant distress or impairment in social, occupational, or other important functions. It should not appear exclusively during the course of another mental or medical disorder, or when alcohol, medication, or other substances are being used.

*Primary hypersomnia*

*Aetiology*

Up to 5% of the population experience hypersomnia at some point in their life, and it is more prevalent in males. The causes can vary widely, but often the symptoms begin before the age of 30 years, and continue to progress unless treated. Some research suggests that sleep disruptions during the night (e.g. breathing-related sleep disorders) result in a lack of REM sleep, so the person feels tired despite the fact that they have slept through the night.

*Symptoms*

The criterion for a diagnosis of primary hypersomnia is excessive sleepiness for at least 1 month, demonstrated by prolonged sleep during the night or excessive daytime sleep. The hypersomnia must cause significant distress or impairment for the individual, and it should not occur exclusively during another mental illness, medical condition, or substance use.

## Narcolepsy

Narcolepsy is diagnosed when a person has repeated sudden occurrences of sleep for a period of at least 3 months. For a diagnosis of narcolepsy to be made, at least one of the following must be present: cataplexy (brief episodes of sudden loss of muscle tone) and REM intrusions (REM sleep occurs at unexpected times and results in hallucinations or sleep paralysis). Symptoms caused by another mental disorder, a medical condition, or substance use must be ruled out.

**Further reading**

Charney PR, Geyer GD and Berry RB. *Clinical Sleep Disorders*. Lippincott Williams & Wilkins: Philadelphia, PA, 2004.
Hirshkowitz M and Smith PB. *Sleep Disorders for Dummies*. For Dummies: New York, 2004.

# Trauma and stress-related disorders

DSM-5 has introduced a new section, 'Trauma and stress-related disorder', so post-traumatic stress disorder (PTSD) is now included within this larger diagnostic framework. This change occurred following a review of the empirical literature, which concluded that PTSD consists of four distinct clusters, rather than the original three clusters in DSM-IV.[10] These clusters contain the following symptoms after a person is exposed psychologically or physically to exceptionally threatening or catastrophic experiences, such as serious injury, sexual or criminal assault, warfare, or natural catastrophe.

- Re-experiencing the event—they have spontaneous memories of the traumatic event, recurrent dreams related to it, flashbacks, or other intense or prolonged psychological distress.
- Heightened arousal—since the event they have exhibited aggressive, reckless, or self-destructive behaviour, or have been experiencing sleep disturbances, hypervigilance, or related problems.
- Avoidance—they are now avoiding circumstances that invoke distressing memories, thoughts, feelings, or reminders of the event.
- Negative thoughts, mood, or feelings—these range from a persistent and distorted sense of blame of self or others, to estrangement from others or markedly diminished interest in activities, to an inability to remember key aspects of the event.

DSM-5 now also contains a separate section for children–this is because children under 8 years of age do not normally complain of PTSD symptoms, but instead often exhibit sleep, behavioural, or concentration problems. PTSD is commonly identified (up to 30%) in children attending Accident and Emergency departments,[11] and therefore children should be asked separately and directly about the presence of these symptoms.

## Typical symptoms

- Repeated reliving of the trauma in intrusive memories, 'flashbacks', or dreams.
- A persistent background sense of 'numbness'.
- Emotional blunting.
- Detachment from other people.
- Lack of responsiveness of the person to their surroundings.
- Anhedonia (failure to enjoy positive emotional experiences).
- Avoidance of activities and situations reminiscent of the trauma.
- Fear and avoidance of cues that remind the person of the original trauma.
- Autonomic hyperarousal with hypervigilance (constantly feeling that something awful is about to happen).
- An enhanced startle reaction.
- Insomnia.
- Anxiety and depression.
- Suicidal ideas.
- Excessive use of alcohol or drugs—this may be a complicating factor.
- Rarely, there may be dramatic, acute bursts of fear, panic, or aggression, triggered by stimuli arousing a sudden recollection and/or re-enactment of the trauma, or of the original reaction to it.

The symptoms of psychosis and PTSD are similar. The flashbacks can be similar to or the same as hallucinations. The intense fear and 're-experiencing' of symptoms in PTSD can be akin to delusions. Both PTSD and psychosis can lead to disturbed sleep patterns, difficulty in concentrating, personal neglect, and withdrawal from others and/or activities. The paranoia that is often associated with psychosis can mirror the hypervigilance that people with PTSD may experience. For this reason, NICE 2014[12] recommends that people with psychosis or schizophrenia should be assessed for PTSD and other reactions to trauma because they are likely to have experienced previous adverse events or trauma associated with the development of the psychosis or as a result of the psychosis itself.

People who have been involved in major disasters, refugees, and asylum seekers can suffer both short- and long-term consequences. Although stand-alone debriefing sessions are not recommended, screening of people involved in such events should be considered by authorities.[11]

## Treatment

- Early intervention and/or watchful waiting. The severity of the initial reactions provides an indication of the need for psychological intervention. If symptoms are mild and have been present for up to 4 weeks after the trauma, watchful waiting is used to monitor and follow up the individual.
- Practical support and social factors, including providing information on symptoms and advice on how to access services, and being responsive to different languages and cultures by providing interpreters and bicultural therapists.
- Psychological CBT intervention.
- Drug treatment (although the evidence for the effectiveness of medication in PTSD is poor).[11]
- Inclusion of families and carers, who have a central role to play in supporting people with PTSD. Depending on the trauma, they may also need help themselves.

## References

10 Friedman M, Resick P, Bryant RA and Brewin CR. Considering PTSD for DSM-5. *Depression and Anxiety* 2011; **28**: 750–69.
11 National Institute for Health and Care Excellence (NICE). *Post-Traumatic Stress Disorder (PTSD): the management of PTSD in adults and children in primary and secondary care.* CG26. NICE: London, 2005. ℘ www.nice.org.uk/guidance/CG26/chapter/1-Guidance
12 National Institute for Health and Care Excellence (NICE). *Psychosis and Schizophrenia in Adults: treatment and management.* CG178. NICE: London, 2014. ℘ www.nice.org.uk/guidance/CG178

## Further reading

Frueh C, Grubaugh A, Elhai JD and Ford JD. *Assessment and Treatment Planning for PTSD.* John Wiley & Sons Inc.: Hoboken, NJ, 2012.
PTSD Alliance. ℘ www.ptsdalliance.org
Semple D and Smyth R (eds). *Oxford Handbook of Psychiatry,* 4th edn. Oxford University Press: Oxford, 2013.
Soli P and Williams MB. *The PTSD Workbook: simple, effective techniques for overcoming traumatic stress symptoms.* New Harbinger Publications, Inc.: Oakland, CA, 2002.

# Other concepts of mental health and illness

The most common and international definition of health was produced by the World Health Organization (WHO) in 1946. They defined health as 'a state of complete physical, mental and social well-being and not merely the absence of disease or infirmity'.[13] This definition of health relates not only to our minds and our bodies, but also to our quality of life—including families, friends, and communities.

Although not without its critics, this definition can also be a starting point for thinking about the concept of mental health. It refers not only to our inner mental well-being, but also to the quality of the way we live our lives.

A concept can be defined as an abstract thought or idea. There is no one concept of mental health, but several categories of approach that have informed the thinking and delivery of mental health and illness care over the years.

## The medical concept

The medical concept was developed by psychiatrists. They believe that illness stems from a chemical imbalance within the brain. The focus of treatment has been on chemical intervention in the form of medication, or on psychosurgery. This concept is often criticized for ignoring social or familial links.

## The anti-psychiatry concept

This concept stems from the work of Thomas Szasz.[14] He proposed that the experiences and behaviours referred to as mental illness were in fact problems associated with living, and with an individual's inability to adapt to the world around them. Although Szasz acknowledged that some behaviour has a physical cause, such as acquired brain injury, he concluded that psychiatrists are oppressors and that there is no such thing as mental illness. He has been criticized for ignoring the genuine suffering of people with mental illness.

## The family concept

RD Laing[15] contributed to this debate, and maintained that the family was the cause of mental illness, particularly schizophrenia. He regarded the family as a pathogenic institution that was unable to provide a consistent approach for a child. As a result, the child would grow up unable to please their parents and suffering intolerable emotional stress, leading to mental illness. He proposed that psychiatrists collude with the family in an attempt to control behaviour that others consider a nuisance.

## The labelling concept

Also in the 1960s, it was proposed by Thomas Scheff[16] that labelling was the single most important cause of mental illness, in that a person would become what they were labelled. He believed that certain bizarre or 'deviant' behaviours which did not fit into a defined category such as 'Teddy boy' or 'Mod' (later examples might be 'punk rocker' or 'Goth') were labelled as mentally ill. As a consequence, psychiatric symptoms can be seen as instances of residual deviancy which have become part of society's cultural stereotype of mental illness.

This concept helped to draw attention to the notion of stigmatization of the mentally ill, although Scheff was criticized on the grounds that the majority of people who become psychiatric patients suffer serious mental disturbances before any label is applied to them.

## Psychoanalytical concepts

There are many and varied concepts in this category that understand the individual from the perspective of their unconscious and their early childhood experience. Freud's psychodynamic structure of personality suggests that behaviour is influenced by the id, the ego, and the superego. We are born in the id and our personality develops in stages during childhood. If there are conflicts associated with a particular phase of personality development (oral, anal, phallic, latent, and genital), fixations can develop that become manifested in personality. Jung and Erikson developed the broader psychodynamic approach, maintaining that it is the social world that influences personality development.

Other concepts include attachment theory, which explores the impact of early relationships with the primary carer (typically the mother). The bond between mother and child, or the lack of it, is thought to have an impact on the child's ability to engage with the world. At the heart of the theory lies a paradox in that children who form very close attachments to their mother are also most able to express their independence. Freudian concepts suggested that failure to break these attachments results in emotional trauma that could lead to later mental illness.

## References

13 World Health Organization. *Constitution*. WHO: Geneva, 1964.
14 Szasz T. *The Myth of Mental Illness*. Harper: New York, 1961.
15 Laing RD and Easterton A. *Sanity, Madness and the Family: families of schizophrenics*. Tavistock: London, 1964.
16 Scheff T. *Being Mentally Ill: a sociological theory*. Aldine: Chicago, IL, 1966.

## Further reading (the classics)

Bental R. *Madness Explained: psychosis and human nature*. Penguin Books: London, 2004.
Gabbard G, Beck JS and Holmes J. *Oxford Textbook of Psychotherapy*. Oxford University Press: Oxford, 2005.
Holmes J. *John Bowlby and Attachment Theory*. Routledge: London, 1993.
Pilgrim D. *Key Concepts in Mental Health*. Sage Publications: London, 2005.

# UK mental health legislation

**Patrick Callaghan**

**Patricia McBride**

**Patrick Callaghan**

# Mental Health Act 2007

The detention of patients into mental health services is governed by the Mental Health Act (England and Wales) 2007. The Mental Health Act (MHA) 2007 is essentially an amendment to the MHA 1983. Table 8.1 outlines the main provisions of the MHA 2007.

Table 8.1 Mental Health Act 2007: main provisions

| Section number and purpose | Maximum duration | Can patient apply to MHRT? | Is there an automatic MHRT hearing? | Can nearest relative apply to MHRT? | Do consent to treatment issues apply? |
|---|---|---|---|---|---|
| 2 Admission for assessment: application may be made by the nearest relative or an approved mental health professional (AMHP), and supported by two medical recommendations | 28 days, not renewable | Within first 14 days | No | No | Yes |
| 3 Admission for treatment: application may be made by the nearest relative or an AMHP, supported by two medical recommendations | 6 months. May be renewed for 6 months, then annually | Within first 6 months, then in each period | Yes, at 6 months, then every 3 years (yearly if under 16 years of age) if no application | No | Yes |
| 4 Emergency admission for assessment made by at least one medical recommendation | 72 hours. Not renewable, but a second medical recommendation can change to s2 | Yes, but only if s4 is converted to s2 | No | No | No |
| 5(2) Doctor's or approved clinician's holding power | 72 hours. Not renewable | No | No | No | No |
| 5(4) Nurse's holding power | 6 hours. Not renewable, but a doctor or approved clinician can change to 5(2) | No | No | No | No |

(continued)

**Table 8.1** (Contd)

| Section number and purpose | Maximum duration | Can patient apply to MHRT? | Is there an automatic MHRT hearing? | Can nearest relative apply to MHRT? | Do consent to treatment issues apply? |
|---|---|---|---|---|---|
| 7 Reception in guardianship | 6 months<br>May be renewed for 6 months, then yearly | Within first 6 months, then in each period | No | No | No |
| 16 Doctor re-classifies the mental disorder | For the duration of the detention | Within 28 days of being informed | No | No | No |
| 18 Transfer from guardianship to hospital | 6 months<br>May be renewed for 6 months, then annually | Within first 6 months, then in each period | Yes, at 6 months, then every 3 years (yearly if under 16 years of age) if no application | No | Yes |
| 17 Supervised community treatment (SCT): provisions for people to be discharged from inpatient detention under a Community Treatment Order (CTO) | 6 months, may be renewed for 6 months, then annually | Within first 6 months, then in each period | Yes, at 6 months, then every 3 years | Yes | Yes |
| 25 Restriction of discharge by nearest relative | Variable | No | No | Within 28 days of being informed | No |
| 135 Warrant to search for and remove patient | 72 hours<br>Not renewable | No | No | No | No |
| 136 Police power in public places to remove person to a place of safety | 72 hours<br>Not renewable | No | No | No | No |

MHRT, Mental Health Review Tribunal; AMHP, approved mental health professional.

**Further reading**

Department of Health. *Guide to the Mental Health Act 1983*. Department of Health: London, 2008.
Jones R. *The Mental Health Act Manual*, 11th edn. Sweet & Maxwell: London, 2007.

# Mental Health Act 2007: key changes from the Mental Health Act 1983

### Definition of mental disorder
A single definition applies throughout the act; for the purposes of the Act a mental disorder is 'any disorder or disability of the mind'.[1]

### Criteria for detention
People cannot be compulsorily detained unless appropriate medical treatment is available.

### Professional roles
The group of professionals who are able to take on the functions of the approved social worker (ASW) and responsible medical officer (RMO) is expanded to include registered mental health nurses, registered learning disability nurses, registered occupational therapists, and chartered psychologists who hold a relevant practising certificate issued by the British Psychological Society.

### Nearest relative
Patients can apply to a County Court to displace a nearest relative. The County Court can also displace a nearest relative it judges to be unsuitable, and civil partners can be named as nearest relatives.

### Supervised community treatment (SCT)
It allows for SCT for patients detained in hospital to be discharged on a Community Treatment Order (CTO); the patient remains in detention, but lives in the 'community'.

### Electroconvulsive therapy
New safeguards are introduced.

### Tribunals
It reduces the period after which hospital managers must refer patients to tribunals if they do not themselves apply.

### Advocacy
An appropriate national authority will have a duty to provide support to independent advocates.

### Age-appropriate services
Hospital managers must ensure that patients under 18 years are treated in a setting suitable for their age.

### Reference
1 Jones R. *The Mental Health Act Manual*, 11th edn. Sweet & Maxwell: London, 2007.

# Section 5(2): the doctor's or approved clinician's holding power

## The use of Section 5(2)

Section 5(2) grants a doctor or approved clinician the power to detain a voluntary patient if the clinician believes that the patient needs to be assessed for detention under Section 2 or 3. The patient can be detained for up to 72 hours, and it is not renewable.

## Issues for the doctor or approved clinician to consider

- The period of detention starts at the moment when the doctor or approved clinician furnishes the report to the hospital managers.
- The power cannot be used on a patient attending an outpatient clinic.
- Section 5(2) should only be used if all other attempts to assess the person for detention under the MHA have been exhausted at that point.
- A doctor or approved clinician may nominate a (competent) deputy to exercise their functions under Section 5(2).
- Deputies can be nominated by title.
- The hospital managers must let the ward staff know who is the nominated deputy.
- A Section 5(2) report must not be completed to be used in advance of a voluntary patient wishing to leave.

# Section 5(4): the nurse's holding power

### Introduction

The detention of patients into mental health services falls under the auspices of the Mental Health Act (England & Wales) 2007. This chapter outlines the main provisions of Section 5(4), the nurse's holding power.

### The use of Section 5(4)

Section 5(4) may be used by a registered mental health nurse or a registered nurse trained in caring for people with learning disabilities to detain an informal patient for a *maximum period of 6 hours*, where the detention is necessary for the health and safety of the patient or others, and where it is not possible for the RMO to attend.

### Issues for the nurse to consider when using Section 5(4)

- If Section 5(4) is invoked, the nurse must endeavour to secure the attendance of the RMO as soon as possible so that the patient can be assessed for detention under another section.
- Under Section 5(5) of the MHA the nurse must make a report to management as soon as possible after Section 5(4) is invoked.
- If Section 5(4) is invoked, patients must be informed of their rights under this section as soon as possible thereafter.
- If the RMO detains the patient under Section 5(2), the 72-hour period of this detention starts from the time when the nurse made the report of detention under Section 5(4).
- The nurse can make another report for a further 6 hours' detention if the RMO has not arrived before the end of the 6 hours. However, this is against the spirit of the Act and should be discouraged. It may be possible for the RMO under Section 5(3) to nominate someone else to act on their behalf.
- Patients detained under Section 5(4) cannot be given medication against their will, as this section is not covered by Part 4 of the Act governing consent to treatment issues. It might be possible to justify giving a patient medication under Section 5(4), using common law powers.
- Section 5(4) can only be used where the patient is an inpatient being treated for a mental disorder. It cannot be used on a patient who is being treated in a general hospital for a physical illness who becomes mentally ill.

### Further reading

Dimond BC and Barker FH. *Mental Health Law for Nurses*. Blackwell Science: London, 1996.
Jones R. *The Mental Health Act Manual*, 11th edn. Sweet & Maxwell: London, 2008.

# Sections 135(1) and 135(2)

### Introduction

Section 135 is concerned with the forced entry and removal of a person deemed to be suffering from a mental disorder to a place of safety by a police officer on the order of a Justice of the Peace.

### Section 135(1)

- If a Justice of the Peace deems, from information provided by an approved mental health professional (AMHP) under oath, that a person believed to be suffering from a mental disorder is unable to care for him- or herself, or is being ill-treated or neglected, the Justice can issue a warrant authorizing any police officer to remove that person to a place of safety so that an application for detention under Part 2 of the MHA can be considered, or other arrangements for the care of the said individual can be considered.
- If admission to premises where a person thought to be suffering from a mental disorder resides is refused by that person, a Justice can issue a warrant to any police officer to enter the premises, by force if necessary, and remove the person.
- A person removed by force and taken to a place of safety may be detained there for up to 72 hours.
- In the execution of a warrant to remove a person by force, a police officer shall be accompanied by an AMHP and a registered medical practitioner.

### Section 135(2)

- This subsection allows for a warrant to be issued by a Justice of the Peace to a police officer to enter premises, by force if required, to retake a patient who is *already detained*. This applies to patients on a CTO, those under guardianship, or under the Scottish Mental Health (Care and Treatment) Act 2003, if they have absconded from a place where they are required by law to reside.
- People authorized to retake patients under Section 135(2) are police officers, any officer on the staff of the hospital, any AMHP, any person authorized by the hospital managers, or, in the case of a patient under guardianship, any officer on the staff of the local services authority, or any person authorized by the guardian or local services authority.

### Good practices in the use of Section 135

Paragraph 10.6, p. 73 of the Mental Health Act Code of Practice (COP) states:

> When a warrant issued under section 135(2) is being used, it is good practice for the police officer to be accompanied by a person with authority from the managers of the relevant hospital (or local social services authority (LSSA), if applicable) to take the patient into custody and to take or return them to where they ought to be. For patients on supervised community treatment (SCT) it is good practice for this person to be, if possible, a member of the multi-disciplinary team responsible for the patient's care.

Guidance should be available to AMHPs on how to obtain warrants (COP, Para. 10.7).

Magistrates should satisfy themselves that a warrant is a last resort and that all other (legal) methods of entry have been exhausted (COP, Para. 10.10).

The AMHP or the local social services authority should ensure that transport is on hand to take the person to the place of safety (COP, Para. 10.9).

## Further reading

Department of Health. *Guide to the Mental Health Act 1983*. Department of Health: London, 2008.
Jones R. *The Mental Health Act Manual*, 11th edn. Sweet & Maxwell: London, 2007.

# Consent to treatment

### Introduction

Sections 57–62 of the MHA are concerned with treatment for which consent is required. Section 64G is concerned with urgent (emergency) treatment, and it is this that will be focused on here.

### Section 64G: emergency treatment for patients lacking capacity or competence

In an emergency situation anyone can administer treatment to a patient whom they deem to lack capacity to consent to such treatment, but only in the following conditions:

- 1: The person giving the treatment must believe, reasonably, that the person lacks capacity to consent to it, or lacks competence to consent.
- 2: The treatment must be immediately necessary to save the person's life.
- 3: The treatment will prevent a serious deterioration of the person's illness and does not have irreversible physical or psychological consequences.
- 4: The treatment is necessary to prevent the patient causing harm to him- or herself or others, represents the minimum level of interference, does not have irreversible physical or psychological consequences, and does not involve significant physical hazard.
- 5: Treatment may be forced, but only to prevent harm. However, the force must be proportionate to the patient suffering harm, and the seriousness of the harm.
- 6: If the treatment is ECT, or drugs administered as part of ECT, only 3 and 4 apply.
- 7: Para. 23.25 of the COP states: 'These are the only circumstances in which force may be used to treat SCT patients who object, without recalling them to hospital. This exception is for situations where the patient's interests would be better served by being given urgently needed treatment by force outside hospital rather than being recalled to hospital. This might, for example, be where the situation is so urgent that recall is not realistic, or where taking the patient to hospital would exacerbate their condition, damage their recovery or cause them unnecessary anxiety or suffering. Situations like this should be exceptional.'

### Independent mental health advocate

An Independent Mental Health Advocate (IMHA) is specially trained to help people usually detained under the MHA safeguard their rights. People are eligible for an advocate if they are a 'qualifying patient'. A qualifying patient is someone:

- Detained under section 5(2) or 5(3).
- Under conditionally discharged restrictions.
- Subject to a guardianship order.
- On a supervised community treatment order.
- An informal patient being considered for section 57 or section 58a treatment.

Excellent guidance on the role of an IMHA can be found at the following website ℘ http://www.seap.org.uk/services/independent-mental-health-advocacy/about-independent-mental-health-advocacy.html

## Further reading

Department of Health. *Guide to the Mental Health Act 1983*. Department of Health: London, 2008.
Jones R. *The Mental Health Act Manual*, 11th edn. Sweet & Maxwell: London, 2007.

# Mental Capacity Act 2005

### Introduction

The Mental Capacity Act (MCA) came into force on 1 April 2007. The Act is designed to provide legislation to protect people who may lack capacity to make their own decisions, clarifies who can take these decisions, when they can take them, and how to exercise these functions if required. The Act also allows people to make advance decisions (directives) to plan for when they may lack capacity. The Act does not apply to people aged under 16 years.

### The scope of the MCA

The MCA covers the key decisions about people's property and affairs, health and social care treatment, and decisions about personal care in the event that they lack capacity to make their own decisions.

### The principles of the MCA

Five principles underpin the operation of the execution of the MCA:[2]

- A person must be assumed to have capacity unless it is established that they lack capacity.
- A person is not to be treated as unable to make a decision unless all practicable steps to help them to do so have been taken without success.
- A person is not to be treated as unable to make a decision merely because they make an unwise decision.
- An act done or decision made under this Act for or on behalf of a person who lacks capacity must be done or made in their best interests.
- Before the act is done or the decision is made, consideration must be given to whether the purpose for which it is needed can be as effectively achieved in a way that is less restrictive of the person's rights and freedom of action.

### Definition of lack of capacity within the MCA

- Inability to make a decision regarding a particular matter due to temporary or permanent impairment of, or disturbance in, the functioning of the mind or brain.
- A lack of capacity cannot be established simply by reference to a person's age, appearance, or behaviour, which might lead others to make unwarranted assumptions about capacity.
- Whether a person lacks capacity within the meaning of the MCA must be decided on the balance of probabilities.

### Definition of inability to make decisions within the MCA

- Inability to understand information relevant to the decision.
- Inability to retain information.
- Inability to use or weigh information as part of the process of making the decision.
- Inability to communicate the decision by whatever means.

If a person is able to understand information in a way that is appropriate to their situation (e.g. using simple language, visual aids), *they are not judged as unable to understand the information*, even if they can only retain the information for a short period.

## Definition of best interests within the MCA

Section 4 of the MCA defines best interests.[3] A person who is appointed to determine the best interests of another must, as far as it is possible to do so:

- Take account of that person's past and present wishes, especially if these have been written down, such as in an advance directive when the person had capacity.
- Consider the person's beliefs and values that might have influenced their decision.
- Consider whether the person might regain capacity, and when this might be.
- Take into account all of the relevant circumstances.
- Encourage the person to participate in the decision making
- Take account of or consult the views of others who know the person (e.g. carers, lasting power of attorney, or anyone appointed by a court).

## Deprivation of liberty safeguards (DOLS)

(See also Chapter 15.)

DOLS are an important part of the MCA, and were developed to ensure that vulnerable people living in residential homes, supported living settings, and hospitals are not deprived of their liberty unless this is in their best interests. Vulnerable people are those aged 18 years or over who have a mental health problem, including dementia, and who *do not* have mental capacity to make their own decisions.

Under the MCA a person lacks capacity when they:

- do not understand information given to them
- cannot retain the information long enough to make a decision
- cannot weigh up information and understand the consequences of decisions
- cannot communicate their decision by whatever means available.

Depriving someone of their liberty requires a deprivation of liberty authorization, but this cannot be used with a person unless they lack capacity. DOLS do not apply to someone detained under the MHA.

## The safeguards

These include:

- providing the person with a representative or advocate
- giving the person or their representative the right to challenge legally the deprivation of liberty
- providing a system that allows the DOLS to be reviewed and monitored.

## Examples of deprivation of liberty[4]

- A patient being restrained in order to admit them to hospital.
- Medication[5] being given to a person against their will.
- Staff being in complete control over a patient's care or movements for a long period.
- Staff making all decisions about a patient, including choices about assessments, treatment, and visitors.
- Staff deciding whether a patient can be released into the care of others or to live elsewhere.
- Staff refusing to discharge[6] a patient into the care of others.
- Staff restricting a patient's access to their friends or family.

## The deprivation of liberty authorization process[3]

Once a supervisory body receives a deprivation of liberty application they must arrange an assessment within 21 days that seeks to ensure the conditions for a deprivation of liberty are met. These include:

- Age—check that the person is over 18 years old.
- Mental health—decide whether the person has a mental disorder.
- Mental capacity—ensure that the person lacks capacity.
- Best interests—ensure that the deprivation of liberty is in the person's best interest to safeguard them from harm, or the reasonable likelihood of harm.
- Eligibility—assess whether the person meets the requirement for detention under the MHA. If they do, a deprivation of liberty authorization is not appropriate.
- No refusals—check whether any advance decisions are in place, and also whether the authorization conflicts with decisions made by a court order.

## References

2 Department for Constitutional Affairs. *The Mental Capacity Act 2005*. Department for Constitutional Affairs: London, 2005.

3 Bartlett P and Sandland R. *Mental Health Law: policy and practice*, 3rd edn. Oxford University Press: Oxford, 2007.

4 Alzheimer's Society. *Deprivation of Liberty Safeguards (DoLS)*. www.alzheimers.org.uk/site/scripts/documents_info.php?documentID=1327

5 Alzheimer's Society. *Drugs Used to Relieve Behavioural and Psychological Symptoms in Dementia*. www.alzheimers.org.uk/site/scripts/documents_info.php?documentID=110

6 Alzheimer's Society. *Hospital Discharge*. www.alzheimers.org.uk/site/scripts/documents_info.php?documentID=173

# Assessing mental capacity

### Introduction

When assessing mental capacity, the overriding concern is that a person is assumed to have capacity unless there is intellectual disability, dementia, or other forms of cognitive impairment. The MCA upholds the rights of people who have capacity to make decisions about their care. A lack of capacity cannot be attributed to people whose behaviour is simply eccentric.

### Five principles of the MCA[7]

- Assume capacity.
- Help people to have capacity in all practical ways before deciding that they do not have capacity.
- People are entitled to make unwise decisions.
- Decisions for people without capacity should be in their best interests.
- Decisions for people without capacity should be the least restrictive possible.

Figure 8.1 shows the process to be followed when assessing capacity.
There is a four-point capacity test:

- *Communicate*. Can the person communicate their decision?
- *Understand*. Can they understand the information given to them?
- *Retain*. Can they retain the information given to them?
- *Balance*. Can they balance, weigh up, and use the information?

Some professionals find it difficult to distinguish between the Mental Health Act and the Mental Capacity Act. Figure 8.2 outlines the difference between these acts to help to guide you with regard to which one to use.

### Independent mental capacity advocates

The MCA gives rights to some people who lack capacity to have an Independent Mental Capacity Advocate (IMCA). IMCAs represent the rights of people who are unable to represent themselves and their services are provided by independent organizations. The Office of the Public Guardian has produced excellent guidance on the IMCA service. The guidance can be downloaded from ℘ https://www.gov.uk/government/collections/mental-capacity-act-making-decisions

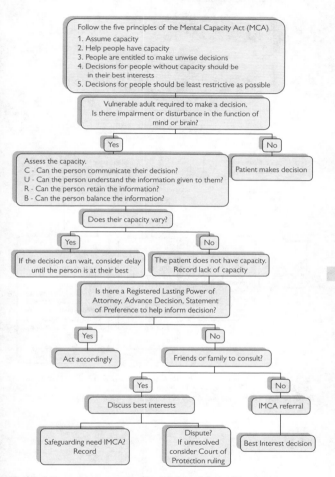

**Fig. 8.1** Guide to assessing capacity. (Royal College of General Practitioners. *RCGP Mental Capacity Act (MCA) Toolkit for Adults in England and Wales 2011.* RCGP: London, 2011.)

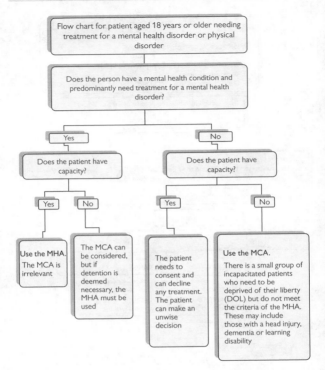

**Fig. 8.2** Relationship between the Mental Capacity Act (2005) and the Mental Health Act (2007). (Royal College of General Practitioners. *RCGP Mental Capacity Act (MCA) Toolkit for Adults in England and Wales 2011*. RCGP: London, 2011.)

### Reference

7 Royal College of General Practitioners. *RCGP Mental Capacity Act (MCA) Toolkit for Adults in England and Wales 2011*. RCGP: London, 2011.

### Further reading

Church M and Watts S. Assessment of mental capacity: a flow chart guide. *Psychiatric Bulletin* 2007; 31: 304–7.

# Mental Health (Care and Treatment) (Scotland) Act 2003

The detention of patients into mental health services in Scotland is governed by the Mental Health (Care and Treatment) (Scotland) Act 2003 (see Table 8.2).

**Table 8.2** Summary of the Mental Health (Care and Treatment) (Scotland) Act 2003

| Section/Part | Duration | Mental Welfare Commission (MWC)/Mental Health Tribunal (MHT) | Appeal | Consent |
|---|---|---|---|---|
| 36 Emergency detention in hospital | 72 hours | MWC informed if mental health officer (MHO) consent is not obtained | No Can be revoked by approved medical practitioner | MHO, where practicable |
| 44 Short-term detention in hospital | 28 days Can be extended by 3 days prior to CTO | MWC/MHT to be informed within 7 days | Patient/ named person can apply to tribunal for revocation of certificate | MHO Named person to be informed |
| 299 Nurse's holding power | 2 hours Can be extended by 1 hour to allow examination to be carried out | MWC to be informed in writing | No | No |
| Part 7 Compulsory Treatment Order (CTO) Treatment enforced either in hospital or in community setting | 6 months, followed by 6 months, then 12-monthly | Tribunal makes decision on application | At time of tribunal hearing and after 3 months | No |

(continued)

**Table 8.2** (*Contd*)

| Section/Part | Duration | Mental Welfare Commission (MWC)/Mental Health Tribunal (MHT) | Appeal | Consent |
|---|---|---|---|---|
| Interim CTO<br>When further assessment is required prior to applying CTO | 28 days, followed by 28 days, maximum 56 days | Tribunal makes decision | At time of tribunal hearing | No |
| 112 Detention in event of failure to attend for treatment under CTO | 6 hours | MHO consulted | No | MHO consent required |
| 130 Assessment of mentally disordered offenders | 28 days | Responsible medical officer (RMO) must report to court before end of 28 days | No | No |
| 133 Compulsion Order<br>For mentally disordered offenders | 6 months, but under regular review by RMO | RMO must report to court if order is no longer appropriate | No | No |
| 134 Detention of acquitted persons for assessment | 6 hours | MWC to be informed within 7 days | No | No |

# The Mental Health (Northern Ireland) Order 1986

### Introduction

This order covers the detention, guardianship, care, and treatment of people subject to detention on account of mental disorder, and applies in Northern Ireland. There are 11 parts to the Order and 137 articles. Here the key articles of the Order that will be of interest to mental health nurses will be described.

### Article 3: definition of mental disorder

Mental disorder is defined as mental illness, mental handicap, and any other disorder or disability of the mind.

### Article 4: criteria for detention

A person may be detained under the Order if the nature or degree of their mental disorder requires detention, and failure to detain would lead to serious physical harm to themselves or others.

### Article 5: application for assessment for admission under the Order

The person's nearest relative or an approved social worker (ASW) may make an application for admission for assessment. A medical recommendation must accompany any application for assessment. Article 6 states that the medical recommendation should come from the person's GP if possible, and the doctor making the recommendation must not be working for the hospital that is admitting the person. The individual making the application for assessment must have seen the person no more than 2 days prior to the date of the application. If an ASW makes the application, they must consult with the person's nearest relative prior to making the application unless, in the opinion of the ASW, this is not practicable or doing so would cause unreasonable delay. If the nearest relative objects to the application for assessment, the ASW must consult with another ASW. If, having consulted with another ASW, the ASW makes the application for assessment, they must record the nearest relative's objection. When a person is admitted following an ASW assessment, the ASW must inform the nearest relative as soon as is practicable following the admission. If a person is admitted following an application by their nearest relative, a social worker must interview the person and provide a report of the person's social circumstances to the responsible medical officer.

### Article 7: assessment of a patient who is already in hospital voluntarily for detention

A patient who is in hospital voluntarily may be detained under the Order by a medical practitioner. In such cases the person's GP, or a doctor with prior knowledge of the patient, must attend the hospital and make a medical recommendation, and an ASW or the patient's nearest relative must make an application for assessment for involuntary detention. In these circumstances the patient can only be detained for a maximum of 48 hours. If it is not possible for a medical practitioner to assess an inpatient for compulsory detention within a reasonable period of time, a registered nurse may detain the patient if they feel it necessary, for a period of up to 6 hours from the time they detain the patient.

## Article 9: period of detention under the Order for assessment

Once a person is admitted under the Order for assessment, they may be detained for 7 days from the date of admission. This detention may be extended for a further 7 days following a report by the responsible medical officer.

## Article 12: period of detention under the Order for treatment

Following the period of admission for assessment, a person may be detained for treatment for up to 6 months from the date of admission. This detention is subject to a report from a medical practitioner appointed by the Mental Health Commission in whose opinion detention is necessary on the grounds that the nature or degree of the patient's mental disorder requires detention for treatment, and failure to detain would lead to serious physical harm to the patient or others. Article 13 allows for renewal of the detention for a further 6 months and then further periods of 1 year.

## Article 18: guardianship

A person aged 16 years or over may be placed into guardianship if they have a mental disorder that warrants guardianship and it is necessary to safeguard them from harm. A guardianship order is founded on two medical recommendations and an ASW recommendation. The application for guardianship can be made by the nearest relative or an ASW, who must have seen the person in the previous 14 days. A guardianship order lasts for 6 months, and may be renewed for a further 6 months, and yearly from then on.

## Articles 42, 43, and 53: persons involved in criminal proceedings

Article 42 allows the courts to remand a person in hospital for 2 weeks for assessment on the basis of one medical opinion. Article 43 allows the courts to remand a person for treatment. Article 53 allows for the transfer of a serving prisoner to hospital for treatment on two medical recommendations on the grounds that the person is suffering from a mental disorder that requires treatment.

## Articles 63, 64, and 68: consent to treatment

Article 63 mandates that detained or voluntary patients may not have neurosurgery unless they consent and the treatment is recommended by a second opinion from an independent doctor. Article 64, which applies only to detained patients, covers other forms of treatment such as ECT, and requires the patient's consent or a second medical opinion. Article 68 allows for urgent treatment in specific emergency cases to be given without the patient's consent or a second medical opinion.

### Articles 70–84: appeals procedures

A person detained under the Order may appeal against this detention to a Mental Health Review Tribunal within 6 months from the date of the original admission. The nearest relative of the detained patient may apply to the Tribunal within 28 days from the date when they are informed that their relative is detained. Any patient who has been detained in hospital for 2 years must be referred by the hospital to the Tribunal. The burden of proof in establishing whether a patient should be discharged from an Order rests with the hospital.

### Further reading

Katona C, Cooper C and Robertson M. Mental health legislation in Northern Ireland. In: *Psychiatry at a Glance*, 4th edn. Blackwell Publishing: London, 2008. pp. 90–1.

The Mental Health (Northern Ireland) Order 1986. Available at  www.legislation.gov.uk/nisi/1986/595

# Safeguarding

### Introduction

In 2006 the UK Government introduced new legislation in the form of the Safeguarding Vulnerable Groups Act 2006. The purpose of the act was to provide for a new Vetting and Barring Scheme for individuals wishing to work with children or vulnerable adults. Before they take up employment with these groups, individuals must be approved by the Independent Safeguarding Authority (ISA). It is against the law for employers to employ people to work with vulnerable groups who are not registered with ISA. Employers can use the Disclosure and Barring Service (DBS) to check whether employees are eligible. An ineligible individual must not take part in any activity with vulnerable individuals that is ISA regulated, and it is a criminal offence for them to do so for any length of time.

### ISA considerations when deciding to register individuals

- Offences: convictions or cautions.
- Evidence of inappropriate behaviour.

### Controlled/regulated activities

- Frequent or intensive support work in general health settings, the NHS, and further education settings.
- People working for specific organizations with frequent access to sensitive records about children and vulnerable adults.
- Support work in adult social care settings.

### Categories of vulnerable groups

Vulnerable adults: a person aged 18 years or older 'is or may be in need of community care services by reason of disability, age or illness; and is or may be unable to take care of him/herself, or unable to protect him or herself against significant harm or exploitation' (UK Select Committee on Health).[8]

### Safeguarding vulnerable adults: the role of the registered nurse[9]

- Identify vulnerable patient groups.
- Describe types of abuse and recognize associated symptoms (see Chapter 6).
- Outline policy and legislation on safeguarding vulnerable adults (see p. 250).

In addition to safeguarding vulnerable adults, registered nurses have an important role in safeguarding children and young people. The nurse's role is outlined in Figure 8.3 and Table 8.3.

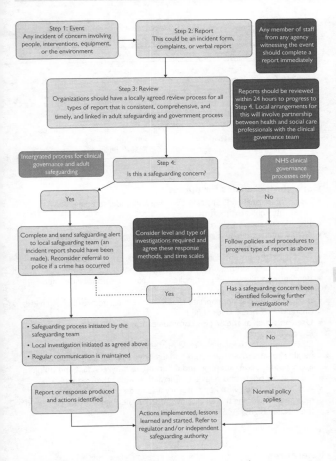

**Fig. 8.3** Clinical governance and adult safeguarding: an integrated process. (Adapted from Department of Health 2010.)

**Table 8.3** The role of the nurse in safeguarding children and young people[10]

| Criterion | Example | |
|---|---|---|
| Identifying a vulnerable child or young person | Linked to gangs | Young carer |
| | Ran away | Looked after by local authorities |
| | Excluded from school | |
| | School refuser | Coerced into criminal activity |
| | Mental health problems | Unaccompanied asylum seeker |
| Signs of harm | Physical abuse | Emotional abuse |
| | Neglect | Sexual abuse |

### Core competencies for nurses[10]

- Use professional and clinical knowledge and understanding of what constitutes child maltreatment.
- Identify any signs of child abuse or neglect.
- Act as an effective advocate for the child or young person, and listen to them.
- Recognize the potential impact of the physical and mental health of a parent or carer on the well-being of a child or young person.
- Be clear about your own and colleagues' roles, responsibilities, and professional boundaries.
- Be able to refer as appropriate to social care if a safeguarding or child protection concern is identified.
- Use tools such as the SAFER communication guidelines[8] to make an effective referral.
- Document safeguarding and child protection concerns in order to be able to inform relevant staff and agencies as necessary. Maintain appropriate record keeping, and differentiate between fact and opinion.
- Share appropriate and relevant information with other teams.
- Act in accordance with key statutory and non-statutory guidance and legislation, including the UN Convention on the Rights of the Child and the Human Rights Act 1998.

### References

8 Department of Health. *SAFER Communication Guidelines*. The Stationery Office: London, 2013. www.gov.uk/government/uploads/system/uploads/attachment_data/file/208132/NHS_Safer_Leaflet_Final.pdf
9 Straughair C. Safeguarding vulnerable adults: the role of the registered nurse. *Nursing Standard* 2011; **25**: 49–56.
10 Royal College of Nursing. *Safeguarding Children and Young People – Every Nurse's Responsibility*. RCN Publishing: London, 2014. www.rcn.org.uk/__data/assets/pdf_file/0004/78583/004542.pdf

### Further reading

HM Government. *The Safeguarding Vulnerable Groups Act (2006)*. The Stationery Office: London, 2006.

# Chapter 9

# Medicines

**Helen Waldock**

**Shameen Mir**

**Neil Brimblecombe**

**Carl Hovey**
Medicines expert/specialist pharmacy advice

# Drugs used in mental health treatment

Medicines used in the treatment of mental health problems fall into four broad categories:

- antipsychotics (neuroleptics)
- antidepressants
- medicines for bipolar disorder
- anxiolytics.

Antipsychotic drugs can be divided into first-generation (typical) and second-generation (atypical) antipsychotics. Most antipsychotics are equally effective at treating psychotic symptoms, with the exception of clozapine, which is more effective than any other antipsychotics. The main differencs between antipsychotics are in their side effect profiles.

## First-generation (typical) antipsychotics

*Examples*

Chlorpromazine, haloperidol, sulpiride, flupentixol, promazine, zuclopen-thixol, and trifluoperazine.

*Actions*

Most act as antagonists at dopamine receptors in the brain. They act predominantly at D2 receptors, but are not selective, so can block all dopamine-receptor subtypes.

*Side effects*

Extrapyramidal side effects (EPSE) include Parkinsonism (including tremor, stiff gait, and mask-like face), dystonia (spasm of a muscle or groups of muscles), akathisia (restlessness), and tardive dyskinesia (late-onset abnormal movements, usually of the hands or parts of the face). Hyperprolactinaemia (raised prolactin levels) may cause reduced sexual libido, impotence in men, and enlarged and painful breasts, lactation, and irregular or no menstruation in women.

## Second-generation (atypical) antipsychotics

*Examples*

Amisulpride, aripiprazole, clozapine, olanzapine, quetiapine, and risperi-done (including the long-acting risperidone injection).

*Actions*

They act as antagonists at a range of dopamine and serotonin receptors, and also at histamine receptors, alpha-adrenoceptors, and muscarinic receptors. Aripiprazole is novel and is a partial antagonist at dopamine receptors.

*Side effects*

In general, EPSE and hyperprolactinaemia are less common than with first-generation antipsychotics. Hyperglycaemia, hyperlipidaemia, diabetes, and weight gain are more common with second-generation antipsychotics.

*Interactions*

Smoking can have a significant impact on the metabolism of clozapine and olanzapine. Lower doses should be considered in non-smokers. Other medicines that prolong the QTc, such as selective serotonin reuptake inhibitors (SSRIs) and high-dose methadone, should be prescribed with caution.

## Antidepressants

According to current guidelines from the National Institute for Health and Care Excellence (NICE), SSRIs are the first-line treatment for depression. Second-line choices include noradrenergic and specific serotonergic antidepressants (NaSSAs), noradrenaline reuptake inhibitors (NARIs), tricyclic antidepressants (TCAs), and serotonin and noradrenaline reuptake inhibitors (SNRIs). The evidence suggests that augmenting an antidepressant with another agent (e.g. another antidepressant or an antipsychotic) is more likely to bring about an improvement in symptoms in more resistant depression than persisting with monotherapy.

### Selective serotonin reuptake inhibitors (SSRIs)

*Examples*
Citalopram, sertraline, fluoxetine, fluvoxamine, and paroxetine. Citalopram has the fewest clinically significant drug interactions, as it is metabolized by many different pathways in the liver.

*Action*
SSRIs selectively block the reuptake of serotonin into nerve cells, thereby increasing the amount of serotonin available in the brain.

### Noradrenergic and specific serotonergic antidepressants (NaSSAs)

*Example*
Mirtazapine.

*Action*
NaSSAs act as an antagonist at the alpha$_2$-adrenoceptors, increasing the central neurotransmission of serotonin and noradrenaline.

### Noradrenaline reuptake inhibitors (NARIs)

*Example*
Reboxetine.

*Action*
NARIs selectively block the reuptake of noradrenaline into nerve cells, thereby increasing the amount of noradrenaline available in the brain. The Medicines and Healthcare products Regulatory Agency (MHRA) and the US Food and Drug Administration (FDA) describe reboxetine as less effective and less suitable for prescribing.

### Serotonin and noradrenaline reuptake inhibitors (SNRIs)

*Examples*
Venlafaxine and duloxetine.

*Action*
SNRIs selectively block the reuptake of both serotonin and noradrenaline into nerve cells, thus increasing the amount of both serotonin and noradrenaline in the brain.

**Tricyclic antidepressants (TCAs)**

*Example*

Lofepramine.

*Action*

TCAs block the reuptake of both serotonin and noradrenaline into nerve cells, thus increasing the amount of both serotonin and noradrenaline in the brain. These drugs also act as antagonists at muscarinic, histaminergic, and alpha-adrenoceptors, which accounts for their side effects.

*Side effects*

Drugs which act to increase serotonin and noradrenaline levels have similar side effects, which include nausea, insomnia, dizziness, and sexual dysfunction. Many of these antidepressants also act as antagonists at muscarinic receptors (particularly TCAs), resulting in blurred vision, dry mouth, and constipation. Hypertension is also a side effect, particularly with venlafaxine. TCAs are particularly cardiotoxic when taken in overdose, and are considered less suitable for prescribing.

**Medicines for bipolar disorder**

*Lithium*

Lithium is primarily used for prophylaxis of bipolar disorder, and is the only medicine that has been shown to reduce suicide rates in those with bipolar disorder. Patients with poor compliance are more likely to relapse than those not taking lithium.

*Action*

Lithium is a naturally occurring ion in the body which exerts its effects in the central nervous system by altering the communication between nerve cells.

*Side effects*

These include gastrointestinal disturbances, fine tremor, weight gain, and hyperthyroidism.

*Common interactions*

Excretion of lithium is reduced, resulting in potential toxicity, by a number of drugs, including diuretics, non-steroidal anti-inflammatory drugs, haloperidol, carbamazepine, SSRIs, angiotensin-converting enzyme inhibitors, angiotensin II-receptor antagonists, and metronidazole.

*Second-generation antipsychotic drugs*

These are the first-line treatment for acute mania and depression in bipolar disorder. They are continued after the acute phase as prophylaxis.

*Examples*

Olanzapine, quetiapine, and risperidone.

*Uses*

They are useful in the treatment of acute episodes of mania and hypomania, and may be used in conjunction with lithium. Olanzapine can be used in the long-term management of bipolar disorder, although this is an unlicensed use.

*Anti-epileptic medicines*

Most of these medicines are used 'off-label'—that is, they do not hold an approved licence for the indication for which they are used. Lamotrigine is effective for the prophylaxis of depressive episodes only. Carbamazepine and valproate are now only used where antipsychotics are ineffective or there has been a previous response to the agent.

*Examples*

Carbamazepine, valproate, and lamotrigine.

*Action*

These medicines act to inhibit sodium ion movement across the membranes of nerve cells in the brain, and to promote the effect of the inhibitory neurotransmitter gamma-aminobutyric acid (GABA). Overall this reduces the excitability of brain tissue.

*Side effects*

Side effects of carbamazepine include nausea, drowsiness, and headache, and those of valproate include dyspepsia, weight gain, fatigue, dizziness, nausea, hair loss, and liver impairment. The use of anti-epileptic medicines in pregnancy is associated with an increased risk of birth defects. Carbamazepine is currently the anti-epileptic of choice in pregnancy.

*Interactions*

Carbamazepine is an inducer of CYP450 liver enzymes, which speed up the metabolism of carbamazepine itself and a number of other medicines, potentially reducing their therapeutic effect.

## Anxiolytics

The first-line treatment for generalized anxiety disorder and panic disorder is an SSRI. Second-line treatment options include alternative SSRIs or an SNRI. Gabapentin should be used as third-line treatment after the first two more effective treatment options have been exhausted. Benzodiazepines should only be used in the short term during crises or during initiation of an SSRI, which can worsen anxiety before it improves.

*Benzodiazepines*

*Examples*

Diazepam, lorazepam, and clonazepam.

*Action*

Benzodiazepines act to enhance transmission of GABA (the inhibitory neurotransmitter) in the brain.

*Side effects*

These include sedation, confusion, addiction, amnesia, headache, and falls in the elderly.

## Further reading

The above prescribing information is not exhaustive, and the following references should be consulted for further information.

Joint Formulary Committee. *British National Formulary (BNF) 67*. Royal Pharmaceutical Society and BMJ: London, 2014. 🔊 https://www.medicinescomplete.com

National Institute for Health and Care Excellence (NICE). *Bipolar Disorder: the management of bipolar disorder in adults, children and adolescents, in primary and secondary care*. CG38. NICE: London, 2006. 🔊 http://guidance.nice.org.uk/CG38/QuickRefGuide/pdf/English

National Institute for Health and Care Excellence (NICE). *Depression in Adults: the treatment and management of depression in adults*. CG90. NICE: London, 2009. 🔊 http://guidance.nice.org.uk/CG90/QuickRefGuide/pdf/English

National Institute for Health and Care Excellence (NICE). Generalised Anxiety Disorder and Panic Disorder (With or Without Agoraphobia) in Adults: management in primary, secondary and community care. CG113. NICE: London, 2011. 🔊 http://guidance.nice.org.uk/CG113/QuickRefGuide/pdf/English

National Institute for Health and Care Excellence (NICE). *Psychosis and Schizophrenia in Adults: treatment and management*. CG178. NICE: London, 2014. 🔊 www.nice.org.uk/guidance/cg178

*Summary of Product Characteristics for Medicines*. 🔊 www.medicines.org.uk

# Safe administration of medicines

The right medicine(s) in the right form must reach the right patient, at the right dose, at the right time, via the right route. One must make the right documentation and monitor the patient for their therapeutic response or development of any side effects. Anything that prevents this may result in a medication error or incident.

## Principles for the administration of medicines

In exercising your professional accountability in the best interests of your patients, you must adhere to the following principles.
- Know the therapeutic use of the medicine to be administered, the indication, normal dosage, side effects, cautions, and contraindications.
- Be certain of the identity of the patient to whom the medicine is to be administered (e.g. check their date of birth). This can be especially difficult in mental health care, as patients do not usually wear identification wrist bands.
- Be aware of the patient's care plan.
- Check that the prescription and the label are clear and unambiguous.
- Check that the prescribed medicines are the same as those listed on the relevant forms (e.g. T2/3, CT11/12, or s62).
- Consider the medicine in the context of the comorbidities of the patient and any coexisting therapies.
- Always consider the dosage, body weight where appropriate, method of administration, route, and timing.
- Check the expiry date of the medicine to be administered.
- Check that the patient is not allergic to the medicine before you administer it.
- Contact the prescriber, or another authorized prescriber, without delay if contraindications to the prescribed medicine are discovered, if the patient develops a reaction to the medicine, or if assessment of the patient indicates that the medicine is no longer suitable for them.
- Make a clear, accurate, and immediate record of all medicines administered, including those intentionally withheld or refused by the patient. Ensure that any written entries and the signature are clear and legible. It is also your responsibility to ensure that a record is made when you delegate the task of administering medicine.
- Where complex calculations are required to ensure that the correct volume or quantity of medication is administered, you are advised to ask a second practitioner to check the calculation independently. This will help to minimize the risk of error.
- If you are supervising a student who is administering medicines, clearly countersign the student's signature.
- You must not administer medication under a patient group direction unless you have been trained and are named under the direction in accordance with local policy.
- You must not administer medicines that require specific training for competence (e.g. intravenous or epidural administration) unless you have received appropriate training and it is up to date.

- The crushing of medicines makes the administration unlicensed. You should contact a pharmacist before doing this if it is in the best interest of the patient, to ensure that there is no other way of administering the medicine, and to check that it is safe to do this.
- Hiding medicines in food or drink is not best practice. However, there may be instances when the patient lacks capacity and it is in their best interest to do this. The decision to conceal medicines in this way must be made in accordance with the Mental Capacity Act.
- You must not take a verbal order for the administration of medicine. Always request written documentation confirming an administration order.

## Management of medicine-related incidents

- A medicine-related incident occurs when something prevents the right patient receiving the right medicine(s) in the right form, at the right dose, at the right time, via the right route.
- If you make an error you must take any action necessary to prevent any potential harm to the patient.
- Any incident must be reported immediately to the prescriber, line manager, or employer, and you must document your actions.
- Most organizations will have an incident-reporting procedure, and this must be followed.
- Make sure that the patient is safe—carry out all necessary observations.
- You should provide a written statement and also complete a Trust incident form. The error must be documented on the drug chart and in the medical and nursing notes.
- Inform the patient of the incident.
- Ensure that actions are taken to prevent the incident from happening again.
- Near misses, or events that occur that could have led to an error, should also be reported. Organizations that are vigilant about reporting low-level-harm incidents and near misses are known to be safe, learning organizations.

## Further reading

NHS Professionals. *CG3 Guidelines for the Administration of Medicines*. NHS Professionals: Watford, 2013. ℘ www.nhsprofessionals.nhs.uk/download/comms/cg3%20-%20administration%20of%20medicine%20guidelines%20v4%20march%202013.pdf

Nursing and Midwifery Council. *Standards for Medicine Management*. Nursing and Midwifery Council: London, 2007. ℘ www.nmc-uk.org/Documents/NMC-Publications/NMC-Standards-for-medicines-management.pdf

# Prescribing medicines

### General principles

- Medicines must be prescribed either by a medical practitioner or by a non-medical prescriber.
- Non-medical prescribers (e.g. nurses, pharmacists, physiotherapists, podiatrists, radiographers) can be independent or supplementary prescribers.
- Independent non-medical prescribers (nurses, pharmacists, physiotherapists, and podiatrists) are able to diagnose conditions and prescribe appropriately within their area of competence.
- Supplementary non-medical prescribers can prescribe any medicine listed within a patient-specific clinical management plan. In this instance it is the independent prescriber (who must be a doctor or dentist) who is responsible for the diagnosis.
- The prescribing of medicines should be based, whenever possible, on the patient's informed consent and their awareness of the purpose of the treatment.
- The prescriber must always check whether the patient has a medicine allergy or is unable to tolerate the medicine to be prescribed.
- Prescribers are responsible for ensuring that the physical monitoring and review recommendations are specified.
- Prescribers should clearly document their prescribing rationale and care plan in the patient's notes.
- The patient should be involved in the choice of their medicine, and should be offered appropriate information about their treatment.
- Where there is a requirement under the Mental Health Act for consent to be given concerning treatment, there should be a valid form reflecting the medicine being administered.

### Inpatients

*The prescription*

Inpatient prescription charts are not legal prescriptions and do not have to conform to the legal requirements, as they are deemed to be a 'hospital order.' However, most organizations treat them as if they were a legal prescription, and as such follow the requirements.

All prescriptions should:
- be clearly written, typed, or computer-generated, and be indelible
- be dated
- state the name and address of the patient
- clearly specify the name of the preparation to be administered (do not use abbreviations)
- clearly specify the quantity to be prescribed
- clearly specify the dose and dose frequency
- be signed in ink by the authorized prescriber
- preferably give directions for use in English

- preferably give the age and date of birth of the patient (this is a legal requirement for prescription-only medicines prescribed for children under the age of 12 years)
- avoid the unnecessary use of decimal points (e.g. 500 micrograms, not 0.5 mg), and if a decimal point is used it should always be preceded by a number.

*Controlled drugs*

A prescription for controlled drugs must also meet the following requirements:

- It must specify the address of the person issuing it.
- In the case of preparations, their form and, where appropriate, their strength must be specified. This can be either the total quantity of the preparation (in both words and figures), or the number (in both words and figures) of dosage units, as appropriate.
- In any other case, the total quantity (in both words and figures) of the controlled drug to be supplied must be specified.
- If a prescription is for a total quantity intended to be dispensed by instalments, it must contain a direction specifying the amount of the instalments which may be dispensed and the intervals to be observed when dispensing.
- If the prescription is issued by a dentist, it should state 'for dental treatment only'.

**Further reading**

Royal Pharmaceutical Society. Medicines, Ethics and Practice: the professional guide for pharmacists. Edition 37. Pharmaceutical Press: London, 2013.

# Assessing and managing the side effects of medicines

## Antidepressants: SSRIs

*Nausea*
- Assessment—direct questioning or observation (e.g. patient may not feel like eating).
- Management—take medicine with food. If the nausea persists, use an anti-emetic.

*Anxiety*
- Assessment—direct questioning and visual observation.
- Management—if the patient is already anxious, start antidepressants at half the usual starting dose, and increase the dose gradually. If the anxiety is severe, a short course of benzodiazepines can be prescribed.

*Sexual dysfunction*
- Assessment—direct questioning (e.g. about difficulty in reaching orgasm).
- Management—this is difficult to manage and usually requires a change of medication (e.g. mirtazapine, moclobemide, reboxetine).

## Antidepressants: TCAs

*Dry mouth*
- Assessment—direct questioning and observation (e.g. fluid consumption).
- Management—this side effect may wear off with time. Reduce the dose where possible. Advise the patient to suck sugar-free sweets, and sip water (but avoid sugary drinks). If the side effect persists, use artificial saliva, or switch to a different antidepressant with fewer anticholinergic side effects, such as an SSRI. A persistent dry mouth can lead to an increase in dental caries.

*Blurred vision*
- Assessment—direct questioning.
- Management—this side effect may wear off with time. Reduce the dose where possible. If the side effect persists, switch to a different antidepressant with fewer anticholinergic side effects, such as an SSRI. Blurred vision cannot be corrected with optical glasses.

*Constipation*
- Assessment—direct questioning and observation of bowel motion.
- Management—dose reduction where possible. If constipation is severe, treat with laxatives. Chronic constipation can lead to faecal impaction, which can be life-threatening. If the side effect persists, switch to a different antidepressant, such as an SSRI.

*Dizziness*
- Assessment—direct questioning, check postural drop.
- Management—this side effect may wear off with time. Reduce the dose where possible. If it persists, switch to an antidepressant with fewer anticholinergic side effects, such as an SSRI. Use this medicine with caution in elderly patients, because of the danger of falls.

## Antipsychotics

*Extrapyramidal side effects*

Assessment can be done both by observation, and more formally, using one of the following rating scales:
- Simpson Angus Scale (SAS)—for drug-induced, acute extrapyramidal side effects. It measures rigidity, tremor, and pooling of saliva in the mouth.
- Barnes Akathisia Scale (BAS)—for drug-induced akathisia.
- Abnormal Involuntary Movement Scale (AIMS)—for tardive dyskinesia and other abnormal involuntary movements associated with antipsychotic drugs.

*Management of extrapyramidal side effects*
- Dystonia—dose reduction, anticholinergic drugs. If it is severe or persistent, consider changing to an atypical antipsychotic.
- Parkinsonism—dose reduction, anticholinergic drug. If it is severe or persistent, consider changing to an atypical antipsychotic.
- Akathisia—dose reduction. Propranolol may be useful. If it is severe or persistent, consider changing to an atypical antipsychotic.
- Tardive dyskinesia—this is difficult to manage. Consider switching to an atypical antipsychotic such as clozapine or olanzapine. The symptoms often get worse before they improve on reducing or stopping the offending agent.

*Prolactin-related side effects*
- Assessment—direct questioning. There may be reduced sexual libido, impotence in men, and enlarged and painful breasts (gynaecomastia), lactation, and irregular or no menstruation in women.
- Management—these side effects may respond to dose reduction. Switch to an atypical antipsychotic, such as olanzapine, quetiapine, or aripiprazole.

*Weight gain*
- Assessment—measurement of baseline weight and subsequent monitoring.
- Management—diet and exercise programmes. Switching antipsychotics may be beneficial.

*Diabetes*
- Assessment—measurement of baseline fasting plasma glucose levels and subsequent monitoring.
- Management—switch antipsychotics (e.g. to amisulpride or aripiprazole). It is possible to continue treatment and treat the diabetes. Consider the risks and benefits in consultation with the patient.

*Dry mouth, blurred vision, and constipation*
- See 'Antidepressants: TCAs' on p. 264.
- Constipation caused by clozapine can lead to faecal impaction, which can be life-threatening.

*Sedation*

This can happen with twice-daily dosing. If daytime sedation is a problem, consider giving all or a larger proportion of the dose at night.

⮞ Electroconvulsive therapy, p. 142.
⮞ People with a mood disorder, p. 86.
⮞ Schizophrenia, p. 186.
⮞ Depression, p. 190.

**Further reading**

Taylor D, Paton C and Kapur S. *The Maudsley Prescribing Guidelines in Psychiatry*, 11th edn. Wiley-Blackwell: Chichester, 2012.

# Nurse prescribing

Nurse prescribing is a major professional development. In May 2006, legislation in England was changed to enable appropriately qualified nurses to independently prescribe, within their area of competence, from the full *British National Formulary (BNF)*. This action provided a direct solution to the need for urgent access to medicines out of office hours, or for discharge processes, and has cut patient waiting times. Research into nurse prescribing suggests that there are high levels of patient satisfaction and no difference from doctors' prescribing methods. Nurse prescribers[1] tend to work in primary and community settings. However, the role is expanding to include inpatient settings. In March 2010, the NHS Prescription Service (NPS) reported that 12.8 million items were prescribed by nurses.[2]

## Educational preparation

To become a nurse prescriber, nurses must undertake a Nursing and Midwifery Council (NMC)-accredited course. Since 2006, nurses who pass the course have been able to prescribe independently, as well as in a supplementary capacity. The duration of the course varies across the UK regions, but generally it consists of 26 days of theory and 12 days of supervised learning in practice with a doctor. Mental health nurses must be supervised by consultant psychiatrists throughout their clinical placement regardless of the setting, as general practitioners do not have the expertise necessary for prescribing psychiatric medication. Many employing organizations arrange additional training to ensure competence in prescribing psychotropic medication (e.g. psychopharmacology modules).

## Types of nurse prescribing

Nurses with a prescribing qualification can act either as a supplementary prescriber for any medication, or as an independent prescriber for any licensed medication except for controlled drugs. Nurses only prescribe for areas in which they are competent.

### Supplementary prescribing

This is a voluntary relationship between an independent prescriber (usually a doctor, although they could be a nurse practitioner) and the supplementary prescriber (the nurse), to implement an agreed clinical management plan (CMP) with the service user's agreement. The nurse can prescribe within the parameters of the CMP, which must state the conditions under which the medication can be changed or altered.

Key factors necessary for supplementary prescribing include:
- communication between prescribing partners
- access to shared patient records (e.g. the Care Programme Approach)
- the service user as an equal partner in their care.

### Independent prescribing

This is where the nurse practitioner takes responsibility for the clinical assessment of the service user, establishing a diagnosis and the clinical management required, as well as taking responsibility for prescribing where necessary.

## Utilizing nurse prescribing

In order to prescribe safely and effectively, nurse prescribers need:

- ongoing supervision
- to use their qualification for the benefit of service users
- opportunities to prescribe, and policies to support prescribing, including access to a budget
- to maintain competence in line with the national frameworks
- to work within the local reporting and recording policies and protocols.

## References

1 Jones K, Edwards M and While A. Nurse prescribing roles in acute care: an evaluative case study. *Journal of Advanced Nursing* 2011; **67**: 117–26.
2 NHS Prescription Services. *Update on Growth in Prescription Volume and Cost in the Year to March 2010.* ℘ www.nhsbsa.nhs.uk/PrescriptionServices/Documents/Volume_and_cost_year_to_Mar_2010.pdf

## Further reading

Jones A. *Nurse Prescribing in Mental Health.* John Wiley & Sons: Chichester, 2009.

# Culture

**Patrick Callaghan**

**Edward McCann**

# Culturally capable mental health nursing

Mental health nurses play an important part in delivering equality in mental health services, through culturally capable practice. However, there is widespread evidence that people from black and minority ethnic (BME) groups do not feel that the care they receive is equal, equitable, and sensitive to their needs.

## What is culture?

Culture is a shared set of learned behaviours, values, beliefs, norms, assumptions, perceptions, customs, social interactions, and the world view of a particular group.[1]

## What is cultural capability?

- *Awareness and respect*[1] for the ideas, beliefs, values, customs, expressions, and world view of people from different races, ethnicities, and cultures.
- *Willingness* to work towards achieving capability.
- *Ability* to see each person as an individual with needs, desires, and aspirations that may be moulded by their culture, race, or ethnicity.

## Framework of values for mental health and race equality

The National Institute for Mental Health in England had identified the following framework of values for mental health practice:

- recognition of the role of values in all areas of practice
- raising awareness of the values involved in different situations and how they affect practice
- respect for the diversity of service users' values
- respect for diversity within mental health care that is service user-centred, recovery oriented, and multidisciplinary.

## Values underlying cultural capability

- *Awareness*[1] of your own value base, level of comfort with diversity, and personal biases.
- *Acceptance* of difference (knowing that it does not mean inferiority), accepting your own and others' limitations, learning from others, and making amends when necessary.
- *Knowledge*—the need to be learning at all times, and the need to increase your knowledge of diversity.
- *Flexibility* in handling unexpected situations.

## The role of the culturally capable mental health nurse

- Increase your own multicultural understanding, and be aware of your own biases.
- Assess the extent to which people are oriented to their culture (i.e. not all people belonging to the same ethnic group will be oriented to the same culture).
- Explore and assess how culture relates to thoughts, feelings, and behaviour.

- Demonstrate cultural sensitivity through understanding different experiences.
- Respect cultural norms in communication styles.
- Be aware of and avoid stereotyping.
- Ask, listen, and respect.
- Be flexible, and accommodate individual needs as far as possible.
- Respect and accept diversity.

→ Transcultural mental health nursing, p. 24.

## Reference

1 Allot P. *Celebrating Cultural Diversity: developing cultural capability*. National Institute for Mental Health in England, University of Wolverhampton: Wolverhampton, 2005.

## Further reading

Department of Health. *Delivering Race Equality in Mental Health Care: an action plan for reform inside and outside services*. Department of Health: London, 2005. Available at ℘ www.dh.gov.uk

# Working with people from different cultural and ethnic groups

Mental health nurses often work in multicultural settings and interact with people from different cultural and ethnic groups. People within these groups often behave and communicate in different ways.

## Communication issues

When working with people from different cultural and ethnic groups, communication problems may arise due to:

- *rules*—groups have different rules for communication
- *language*—different groups often have their own language and dialect
- *motivation*—factors that drive communication, such as rules and rituals, may vary
- *ideals and values*—different beliefs underpin communication
- *cooperation and competition*—communication may be driven by these goals
- *collectivism and individualism*—communication may be directed at promoting the collective or the individual good
- *greetings and other rituals*—different groups have different rituals and ways of greeting each other (e.g. handshakes, kissing).

## Communication styles

Different cultural and ethnic groups have different styles of communication. The following issues may arise.

- Cultural context of language—the influence of culture on language varies.
- Self-disclosure—the meaning, use, and nature of self-disclosure vary between different groups.
- The preservation of face (i.e. not humiliating someone in front of others) is particularly important in certain groups (e.g. Chinese and Japanese people).
- The use and meaning of silence vary in different cultures.
- The level of respect for truthfulness varies in different cultures.
- Complimenting and responding to compliments may take different forms in different cultures.
- Non-verbal behaviour has different meanings in different cultures.

## The role of the mental health nurse

- Increase your own multicultural understanding, and be aware of your own biases.
- Assess the extent to which people are oriented to their culture (i.e. not all people belonging to the same ethnic group will be oriented to the same culture).
- Explore and assess how culture relates to thoughts, feelings, and behaviour.
- Demonstrate cultural sensitivity through understanding different experiences.
- Respect cultural norms in communication styles.
- Beware of and avoid stereotyping.

- Ask, listen, and respect.
- Avoid using partners or children as interpreters. In many cultures it is unacceptable to talk about intimate matters in front of family members.
- Be flexible, and try to accommodate individual needs as far as possible.

→ Transcultural mental health nursing, p. 24.

## Further reading

Department of Health. *Delivering Race Equality in Mental Health Care: an action plan for reform inside and outside services.* Department of Health: London, 2005. Available at ✆ www.dh.gov.uk

Fernando S. *Cultural Diversity, Mental Health and Psychiatry: the struggle against racism.* Brunner-Routledge: Hove, 2003.

# Sexuality and mental health: a research study

The area of sexuality and people with mental health problems is under-researched, with only one study giving direct guidance to mental health nurses.

## Study aims

In 2010, a study by McCann[2] aimed to identify sexual and relationship needs as perceived by users of mental health services who were living in the community. The objective of this mixed methods study was to discover service users' past and present sexual experiences and to elicit their hopes and aspirations for the future. Potential obstacles to sexual expression were highlighted through an exploration of subjective experiences of the issues that were important to service users.

## Sample and context

A total of 30 people with a medical diagnosis of schizophrenia agreed to be interviewed at a clinic in North London, where they regularly attended to receive depot medication.

## Data collection

Data were collected through:
- a questionnaire relating to demographic characteristics
- an interview schedule incorporating the determinant factors of sexual behaviour through life[3]
- relevant sections of the Camberwell Assessment of Need[4]
- a semi-structured interview designed specifically for the study.

## Analysis

Computer software packages were used to analyse both the quantitative and the qualitative data.

## Findings

The findings revealed that the service users had clear ideas about what constituted a fulfilling intimate relationship. The majority of the participants identified sex and relationship needs, and aspired to have relationships in the future. Obstacles were highlighted, which included medication issues, body image, stigma and discrimination, support and the opportunity to discuss concerns, and access to family planning services or sexual and relationship therapy. The service users seemed comfortable about sharing details of their intimate experiences during the interviews, none of which had to be prematurely terminated. A model of psychosexual care was proposed that includes rigorous methods of engagement, assessment, intervention, and evaluation.

## The role of the mental health nurse

Discussion of thoughts, feelings, and beliefs in relation to sexual aspects of health care is a challenging feature of nursing practice that requires sensitivity, confidence, a shared language, understanding, and care. It presents other challenges in terms of education and professional role development, such as addressing inadequate knowledge of sexuality, exploring and modifying negative attitudes to sexuality, reducing discomfort with sexuality, and examining perceptions about the legitimacy of sexuality within nursing roles.

## References

2  McCann E. Investigating mental health service user views regarding sexual and relationship issues. *Journal of Psychiatric and Mental Health Nursing* 2010; **17**: 251–9.

3  Pfeiffer R and Davis G. Determinants of sexual behaviour in middle and old age. *Journal of the American Geriatric Society* 1972; **20**: 151–8.

4  Slade M et al. *Camberwell Assessment of Need*. Gaskell: London, 1999.

# Sexuality (sexual orientation) and mental health

Sexual orientation refers to the sex, sexes, gender, or genders to which a person is attracted and which form the focus of a person's loving or erotic desires, fantasies, and natural feelings. Other terms such as 'sexual preference' and 'sexual inclination' have related meanings. Some believe that sexuality is fixed early in life, while others believe that it is fluid and reflects preference and choice. The term 'sexual orientation' may also refer to the 'individuality' of a person, either by choice or as an expression of an inner attribute.

The majority of mental health professionals, backed by nearly 40 years of research, believe that it is possible to develop a happy and productive life in the context of a lesbian, bisexual, or gay ('les-bi-gay') sexual orientation, identity, and lifestyle. DSM-IV ceased to list homosexuality as a mental illness. The only diagnostic reference to homosexuality in that edition of the manual relates to 'persistent and marked distress about sexual orientation', and it is the distress that characterizes the disorder, not the orientation itself. The desire to have sex is one of the basic drives of human behaviour.[5]

The NHS Plan and many other NHS drivers for change are committed to a standard of equal access to, and equity of treatment in, health care services. Currently, the experiences of many lesbian, gay, and bisexual service users fall far short of this standard. Mental health workers sometimes fail to acknowledge same-sex partners and their families. Ignoring a service user's partner can result in them not participating in the care of the ill person. It is best practice to involve those closest to the service user, who have knowledge of his or her own wishes.

## Next of kin

There is widespread misunderstanding about the term 'next of kin'. In a health care setting, this term has a very limited legal meaning—it relates to the disposal of a person's belongings to blood relatives, if the person has died intestate. However, the term is also used in a number of other different ways—many service users think it means someone whose relationship to them has legal recognition. Therefore asking for a person's 'next of kin' may confuse them, and is unlikely to give you the information that you need.

For those patients who are detained under the Mental Health Act 2007 (and this is a minority of service users who are receiving help from mental health care providers), the issue of next of kin is often confused with the role of the 'nearest relative'. The role of the 'nearest relative' is to advocate on behalf of a service user. In the past, it has been difficult for same-sex partners to gain recognition as the nearest relative. However, in a recent case brought under the Human Rights Act, a lesbian was successful in gaining recognition for her partner as her nearest relative (a partnership is defined as living with another person as husband or wife for 6 months or longer).

The Civil Partnership (CP) Act became law in December 2005. This act gives same-sex couples the opportunity to legally register their relationship. Once registered, these couples will have similar rights to a heterosexual married couple (in terms of financial and legal matters). For further information, see *Get Hitched! A Guide to Civil Partnerships* (available from ℞ www.stonewall.org.uk).

In 2013 the UK Government published the Marriage (Same Sex Couples) Act 2013 for England and Wales. The key issues can be summarized as follows:

- Marriage of same-sex couples is lawful.
- Members of the clergy may not solemnize same-sex marriage in their church.
- Civil partnership may be converted to marriage under a special procedure at which point the civil partnership is null and void, but the resulting marriage is treated as having existed since the date of the civil partnership.
- Same-sex marriage has the same effect under law as in relation to opposite-sex marriage.

Where a service user is not treated under the Mental Health Act, the same considerations apply as elsewhere in the NHS. There is no limit to who may be selected as the nearest relative or 'next of kin'. The decision should be the service user's choice—it could be their partner or a friend.

The Adults with Incapacity (Scotland) Act 2000 expressly recognizes a same-sex partner as the nearest relative.

➔ Sexual disorders: female, p. 206.
➔ Sexual disorders: male, p. 208.
➔ Sexual disorders: female and male, p. 210.

**Reference**

5 HM Government. *Marriage (Same Sex Couples) Act 2013.* The Stationery Office: London, 2013.

# Older people

**Soo Moore**

# Mental health disorders common in later life

Older people can be subject to a whole range of mental health disorders (➔ Chapter 7), the most common of which are dementia and depression. The Mini Mental State Examination (MMSE) with a combined cognitive assessment is used to support the diagnostic process.[1]

There are a number of different types of dementia, the most common of which is Alzheimer's disease, which accounts for about 60% of cases.

- Alzheimer's disease changes the chemistry and structure of the brain, causing brain cells to die.
- Vascular dementia is caused by strokes or small-vessel disease, which affect the supply of oxygen to the brain.
- Frontotemporal dementia is a rare form of dementia that affects the front of the brain. It includes Pick's disease, but most commonly affects people under 65 years of age.
- Dementia with Lewy bodies is caused by tiny spherical protein deposits that develop inside nerve cells in the brain.

These conditions have the potential to significantly reduce quality of life, dignity, and independence for the older person. Effective assessment and intervention by mental health nurses can make a difference in supporting the older person to be independent and to have a life that is worth living.

## Dementia

The term 'dementia' is descriptive, and covers a global deterioration in mental function due to brain disease. It is progressive and chronic. Deterioration may be seen in:

- memory
- thinking
- orientation
- comprehension
- calculation
- learning capacity
- language
- judgement
- emotional control
- social behaviour
- motivation.

These losses can have a powerful effect upon the person and their family. There is no cure, but effective and timely psychological and physical intervention from nurses—using Triangle of Care[2] principles involving the person with dementia (patient), the staff member, and the carer—can promote safety, support communication, sustain well-being, and help to maintain social networks and relationships.

### Prevalence

The World Alzheimer Report 2013[3] highlights the fact that, as the world population ages, the traditional system of 'informal' care by family, friends, and community will require much greater support. Globally, 13% of people aged 60 years or over require long-term care. Between 2010 and 2050, the total number of older people with care needs will nearly treble, from 101 million to 277 million.[3]

## Depression

Depression in older people has all the characteristics of depression in the general population (→ Depression, p. 190). However, some of the symptoms of depression are more common in older people, while others are less common in this age group.

→ People with a mood disorder, p. 86.

*Symptoms of depression that are more common in old age*
- Complaints related to bodily rather than emotional functioning.
- Loss of or reduced ability to take pleasure in activities.
- Ideas of guilt, worthlessness, death, and suicide.
- Agitation.
- Decline in self-care.
- Deliberate self-harm.
- Suicide.

*Symptoms of depression that are less common in old age*
- Tiredness.
- Sleep disturbance.
- Weight loss.

Depression is treatable. Antidepressant medication, combined with talking therapies such as counselling, group therapy, life review, and social support, usually return the person's mood to normal.

*Prevalence of depression*
In a population of people aged over 65 years, one would expect around 10–15% to exhibit some depressive symptoms, and about 3% to be diagnosed as having severe depression.

## References

1 Petersen RC et al. Practice parameter: early detection of dementia: mild cognitive impairment (an evidence-based review). Report of the Quality Standards Subcommittee of the American Academy of Neurology. *Neurology* 2001; 56: 1133–42.

2 Carers Trust and Royal College of Nursing. *The Triangle of Care. Carers included: a guide to best practice for dementia care.* Carers Trust: London, 2013. ℘ www.rcn.org.uk/__data/assets/pdf_file/0009/549063/Triangle_of_Care_-_Carers_Included_Sept_2013.pdf

3 Alzheimer's Disease International. *World Alzheimer Report 2013. Journey of caring: an analysis of long-term care for dementia.* Alzheimer's Disease International: London, 2013. ℘ www.alz.co.uk/research/world-report-2013

## Further reading

Department of Health. *Living Well with Dementia: a national strategy.* Department of Health: London, 2009.

Jacoby R, Oppenheimer C, Dening T and Thomas A (eds). *Oxford Textbook of Old Age Psychiatry*, 4th edn. Oxford University Press: Oxford, 2008.

# Age-sensitive mental health nursing

Nursing older people with mental health problems requires a complex portfolio of skills, knowledge, motivation, values, and beliefs. Above all, the role requires the nurse to feel and display warmth, genuineness, and respect towards an undervalued group within society.

Working with older people is challenging and complex, as in old age people are more likely to have a multitude of pathologies. For example, a person aged 85 years, besides having dementia, may well have diabetes, hypertension, and arthritis. The effective mental health nurse has to respond to all of these needs.

## Person-centredness

Person-centredness is a concept that is central to dementia practice. Brooker[4] has outlined the following key features of person-centred care:

- Entering the patient's frame of reference—understanding where they are in time and place, and using this as a vehicle to establish a dialogue.
- Non-judgemental acceptance of the uniqueness of the individual—ensuring that actions and non-verbal communication are not patronizing.
- Seeing the person as a whole.
- Having a positive view of human nature.
- Recognizing the importance of feelings and emotions.
- Recognizing the importance of interpersonal relationships.
- Valuing authenticity in relationships—being honest and sincere in interactions with older people.
- A non-directive approach—allowing the older person to make their own decisions.

These features are seen as a basis for structuring the assessment, planning, and delivery of nursing care for older people. They are the underpinning principles of the delivery of health and social care. Principles of care for people with dementia are outlined in guidance from the National Institute for Health and Care Excellence (NICE).[5]

## The context of nursing

The mental health nurse offers a service to older people and their families in a variety of community and inpatient settings.[6] Nurses use a range of therapeutic interventions to enable the older person to be fully engaged in life. While the person still has capacity, advance statements (which allow them to state what they would wish to be done if they should subsequently lose the capacity to decide or to communicate) should be developed.

As dementia worsens and the person becomes more dependent, decisions about sharing information should be made in the context of the Mental Capacity Act 2005 and its Code of Practice.

## References

4  Brooker D. *Person-Centred Dementia Care: making services better*. Jessica Kingsley Publishers: London, 2007.

5  National Institute for Health and Care Excellence (NICE). *Dementia: supporting people with dementia and their carers in health and social care*. CG42. NICE: London, 2006. ℘ www.nice.org.uk/guidance/CG42/chapter/1-Guidance#/#principles-of-care-for-people-with-dementia

6  Royal College of Nursing. *Dementia: commitment to the care of people with dementia in hospital settings*. RCN Publishing: London, 2013. ℘ www.rcn.org.uk/__data/assets/pdf_file/0011/480269/004235.pdf

# Communicating with the older adult

Effective communication is an essential feature of the mental health care of older people. Nurses have to be aware of their verbal and non-verbal communication. Depression, dementia, and sensory impairments often form barriers to effective verbal communication, and the message is more easily conveyed by non-verbal means.

Effective communication with older people can be achieved by adopting the following approach:

- Keep your posture relaxed.
- Move slowly and deliberately when within 1–2 metres of the older person.
- Do not move your hands or arms into an older person's 'personal space'.
- Ensure that you make your presence known before you touch the older person—approaching from behind them and suddenly touching them can cause alarm.
- Aim to have your eyes at the same level as theirs when talking with an older person—crouch or kneel if talking to someone sitting in a wheelchair.
- Keep your voice level, even, and calm.
- Establish how the person wishes to be addressed and then use this name or title in your interactions with them.
- Maintain eye contact while you are talking.
- Use short sentences, repeating key words if necessary.
- Ask only one question at a time.
- Allow the person time to respond.
- Give only one instruction at a time—if you have a complex request break it down into simple steps.
- Check that the person has understood what you have said.
- Ensure that you are demonstrating you are listening by nodding your head and other appropriate responses.
- Ensure that if the person is using a hearing aid it is turned on, in the appropriate ear, and has a working battery.
- Ensure that, if spectacles are worn, the person is wearing their own glasses, the prescription is current, and the spectacles are clean and appropriate (e.g. not wearing reading glasses while eating lunch).

➲ Interpersonal communication, p. 54.

## Further reading

Killick J and Allan K. *Communication and the Care of People with Dementia*. Open University Press: Buckingham, 2001.

# Reality orientation

Reality orientation therapy (ROT) is a psychosocial intervention that aims to reorientate individuals by means of continuous stimulation and repetitive orientation.

## Group approach

Reality orientation is organized using a group of five or six members, with two therapists or group leaders. Simple material is used to stimulate the participants to think about their relationships in order to maintain them. The main topics for discussion are introductions, the time, the date, the weather, and the location. The aim is to help the individual to become oriented with regard to time, place, and person. Once the group has been established it can move on to activities that promote interpersonal relationships—for example, by using humour or reminiscence.

## 24-hour reality orientation

In this approach, rather than rehearsing orienting information in a group setting, the carer uses opportunities in real life during everyday activities or when delivering personal care to repeat or provide information. Activities might include quizzes, games, or newspaper discussions. This is combined with extra aids in the environment, such as large clocks, message boards, colour-coded signing, and furniture arrangements.

## Monitoring

Baseline observations are recorded before commencing reality orientation, and observations are then repeated at regular intervals, so that even quite small improvements can be detected over time.

## Further reading

Holden UP and Woods RT. *Reality Orientation: psychological approaches to the confused elderly.* Churchill Livingstone: Edinburgh, 1995.

# Reminiscence therapy

Reminiscence therapy is a biographical intervention that uses the normal human activity of revisiting past times and events. In a therapeutic setting this is organized in a systematic way, with the aim of stimulating individuals to engage in social interaction. Revisiting former experiences may help to validate people by stimulating positive emotions associated with their past experience.[7]

Reminiscence therapy is usually conducted in residential homes and day centres, as a facilitated group activity. Sessions can be centred around:
- music and sound recordings
- photographs and films
- outings
- practical activities such as cooking or gardening
- storytelling
- taste, touch, and smell
- drawing, painting, and collage
- handling objects, especially artefacts that are symbolic of past times
- drama.

## Reference

7 Woods B et al. *Reminiscence Therapy for Dementia (Review)*. The Cochrane Collaboration. John Wiley & Sons: Chichester, 2009. http://onlinelibrary.wiley.com/doi/10.1002/14651858. CD001120.pub2/pdf

## Further reading

Bornat J (ed). *Reminiscence Reviewed: perspectives, evaluations, achievements*. Open University Press: Buckingham, 1994.

# Validation therapy

Validation therapy offers the confused older person an empathetic listener, a non-judgemental approach, and an acceptance of their reality.

## Reported benefits of validation therapy[8]

- Restoration of self-worth.
- Minimization of the degree to which the patient withdraws from the outside world.
- Promotion of communication and interaction with other people.
- Reduction of stress and anxiety.
- Stimulation of dormant potential.
- Help in resolving unfinished life tasks.
- Facilitation of independent living for as long as possible.

## Essential techniques of validation

- Centring—the caregiver uses techniques to give their full attention to the patient.
- Using non-threatening factual words to build trust.
- Rephrasing—repeating back to the patient the essence of what they have said.
- Polarity—asking the patient to think about worst-case scenarios to relieve their anxiety.
- Imagining the opposite—can lead to the recollection of a familiar solution.
- Reminiscing.
- Maintaining genuine, close eye contact.
- Using ambiguity—exploring ambiguous statements by using open questions and pronouns.
- Using a clear, low, friendly tone of voice.
- Observing and matching the patient's motions and emotions (mirroring).
- Linking the patient's behaviour with their unmet human need.
- Identifying and using the patient's preferred sense for communication (e.g. sight or hearing).

## Memory clinics

Memory clinics or memory assessment services for the early identification and care of people with dementia can break down barriers and reduce stigma in the following ways:

- The fact that they are called 'memory' rather than 'mental health' or 'old age psychiatry' services removes much of the stigma.
- They improve communication.[9]
- They represent a move away from intimidating psychiatric or other hospital settings to a primary care environment.

## Summary

A range of tailored interventions, such as reminiscence therapy, multisensory stimulation, animal-assisted therapy, and exercise, should be available for people with dementia who have depression and/or anxiety.[9]

## References

8  Neal M and Barton Wright P. Validation therapy for dementia. *Cochrane Database of Systematic Reviews* 2003; 3: CD001394.
9  National Institute for Health and Care Excellence (NICE). *Dementia: supporting people with dementia and their carers in health and social care.* CG42. NICE: London, 2006. ◎ www.nice.org.uk/guidance/CG42/chapter/1-Guidance#/#principles-of-care-for-people-with-dementia

# Transformational leadership

Mental health nursing does not take place in a vacuum. To promote patient experience and sustain recovery-based outcomes, nurses must collaborate with other health care professionals, and work alongside managers to support operational systems, as well as in partnership with people using services, and their respective carers. To achieve this paradigm, nurses appreciate leaders who work alongside them, have presence in clinical areas, and are accessible. By contrast, autocratic, arrogant, and unsupportive leaders are perceived as unhelpful, as they create an environment that is not conducive to staff well-being, which in turn affects patients' experience.[1] Mental health nursing should inspire, support, and create the conditions under which people will flourish. For this reason, every nurse at every level needs to demonstrate transformational leadership styles.

James MacGregor Burns, a historian and political scientist, conceptualized transformational leadership as a process in which 'leaders and followers help each other to advance to a higher level of morale and motivation.'[2] This style supports transformation of systems and changes in organizational culture that need to be incorporated throughout the NHS if the lessons of the Francis Inquiries[3] are to be learned and acted upon.[4]

Transformational leaders:
- act with integrity and honesty
- engage staff and service users in decision making
- clarify their own and others' role expectations
- use actual and inferred evidence to implement decisions
- employ sound communication skills using a variety of methods
- inspire, support, nurture, and empower others
- promote the profession and project a positive image with gravitas locally, nationally, and internationally.

## Past British mental health nurse leaders

### Professor Annie Altschul CBE, FRCN (1919–2001)

Annie Altschul, Professor of Nursing at Edinburgh University from 1976 to 1983, pioneered psychiatric nursing research. In the late 1960s her study of nurse–patient interactions in acute psychiatric care became one of the most cited reports in nursing research literature. She explored the complex processes involved in the development of therapeutic relationships, especially in the early stages of care and treatment.[5,6]

### Eileen Skellern (1923–1980)

Eileen Skellern, Chief Nurse at the Maudsley Hospital, London, made an outstanding contribution to the advancement of mental health nursing. She played a leading role in development of the knowledge, skills, and professional contribution of nurses. She was the first nurse to become an Associate of the Royal College of Psychiatrists. One project of particular note was her participation in the 1969 national working party, chaired by Richard Crossman, the then Secretary of State, to review policy on mental 'subnormality' following revelations of malpractice and the inquiry at Ely Hospital, Cardiff.[7,8]

## References

1  Goodrich J and Cornwell J. *The Contribution of Schwartz Center Rounds® to Hospital Culture 2012.* The King's Fund: London, 2012. ℘ www.kingsfund.org.uk/publications/articles/contribution-schwartz-center-rounds-hospital-culture-2012

2  Burns JM. *Leadership.* Harper Perennial: London, 2010.

3  Francis R. *Report of the Mid Staffordshire NHS Foundation Trust Public Inquiry. Volume 3: present and future Annexes.* The Stationery Office: London, 2013. ℘ www.gov.uk/government/uploads/system/uploads/attachment_data/file/279121/0898_iii.pdf

4  The King's Fund. *Patient-Centred Leadership: rediscovering our purpose.* The Kings Fund: London, 2013. ℘ www.kingsfund.org.uk/sites/files/kf/field/field_publication_file/patient-centred-leadership-rediscovering-our-purpose-may13.pdf

5  Nolan P. Annie Altschul's legacy to 20th century British mental health nursing. *Journal of Psychiatric and Mental Health Nursing* 1999; **6**: 267–72.

6  Barker P. Annie Altschul: progressive champion of psychiatric nursing. *The Guardian* 8 January 2002 ℘ www.theguardian.com/society/2002/jan/08/mentalhealth

7  Winship G, Bray J, Repper J and Hinshelwood RD. Collective biography and the legacy of Hildegard Peplau, Annie Altschul and Eileen Skellern; the origins of mental health nursing and its relevance to the current crisis in psychiatry. *Journal of Research in Nursing* 2009; **14**: 505–17.

8  Russell D. *Eileen Skellern: a biographical essay.* ℘ www.skellern.info/russellessay.html

## Further reading

Callaghan P, Playle J and Cooper L. *Mental Health Nursing Skills.* Oxford University Press: Oxford, 2009.

Philips P, Sandford T and Johnson C. *Working in Mental Health: practice and policy in a changing environment.* Routledge: Abingdon, 2012.

# Developing effective teams

Every team, regardless of the wider organizational context in which it sits, will have a unique team dynamic, an identity, and a micro-culture. Although each team will present differently, all teams require some common principles to be applied in order for them to be developed to their maximum potential.

## Important areas to consider

There are three important areas to consider when developing a team. These are:
- the wider organization
- the purpose and business of the team
- the aptitudes, behaviours, experience, and skills contained within the team.

### The wider organization

In order to develop a team, the boundaries and characteristics of the wider organization need to be clearly understood. This provides the framework within which the team needs to work. These are as follows:
- *The culture*—this incorporates the expressed aims and objectives, philosophy, and mission of the organization as a whole. It defines the purpose and value base of the entire enterprise (**→** Culturally capable mental health nursing, p. 272; **→** Working with people from different cultural and ethnic groups, p. 274).
- *The structure*—this includes the systems, hierarchy, and processes or rules that the organization has put into place in order to achieve its overarching purpose.
- *The lived experience*—this consists of the unspoken and unwritten belief systems that actually exist. It also includes the behaviours that are enacted within the organization. Sometimes the lived experience may differ from the more formal philosophies expressed by the wider organization.

### The purpose and business of the team

A successful team will have clarity about the following:
- its goals and purpose
- its agreed common approach to achieving its goals and purpose
- its mutual sense of joint accountability
- its united interdependence where each role and function is reliant on the effective functioning of the team as a whole.

### The aptitudes, behaviours, experience, and skills contained within the team

A team should be more than the sum of its collective parts. A team that is motivated and working well understands how to utilize the skills base of each of its individual members. In order to develop the team as a whole, together with the skills of its individual members, the aptitudes, behaviours, experience, and skills contained within the team need to be fully understood. If teams are to be developed to reach their full potential, the following aspects must be understood.

- Aptitudes for carrying out certain functions may be held by certain individuals. How should a team respond to this? Should the team allow one person to become a specialized resource or should the whole team continue to hone their skills in this area?
- Working in a team environment can be a challenge. Everyday stresses and tensions can lead to hindering and unhelpful behaviours. For a team to develop in a useful manner, hindering and unhelpful behaviours need to be identified and mitigated against.
- All teams will contain a mixture of experience and skills. Most professional teams are assembled with their individuals already fit for purpose. The art of developing a team is to grow skills and experience so that innovation and flexibility are encouraged.

Teams do not work in isolation. To develop an effective team it is important to understand the macro-culture of the wider organization, the goals and purpose of the team, and the ability of the individuals in the team to be efficient and effective.

## Leading effective teams

A team is 'a small group of people with complementary skills committed to a common purpose and a set of specific performance goals.' The way in which a team is led will have a direct impact upon its potential success. An effective leader will require a set of specific skills, which could include any of the following.

### A commitment to people

- Ensuring that the developmental needs of team members are met.
- Utilizing tools such as appraisal, mentoring, coaching, and consistent supervision.
- Ensuring the individual development of team members—this benefits both the individual members and the team.

### Enthusiasm

- Developing a vision that is known by all, and encouraging team members to buy into it.
- Keeping morale high by acknowledging the expertise within the team and ensuring that it is used for everyone's benefit.

### Ability to take responsibility

- Team leaders are tested under pressure.
- A leader's role is to rise to challenges, to ensure that their team services them, and to delegate roles appropriately.

### Ability to give praise and constructive feedback

The ability to give constructive feedback honestly but without inflicting damage or hurt is an important skill, particularly when the message may be difficult for the other person to hear.

One technique that is used is the 'criticism sandwich'. The team leader first highlights what went well, then brings in areas for development, and ends on a positive achievement.

### A commitment to developing the team

All teams will experience change as new members join, additional skills are added, and the goals of the team change.

The ingredients of an effective team are created by the combination of a skilled team leader, willing team members who are supported and developed, and a set of defined and agreed shared goals. This combination is likely to leave team members feeling good about the team to which they belong.

Team building has been described as 'like coaching, but for a group.'[9] Whether team building is soft (e.g. shared meals, sporting events) or hard (e.g. inter-team learning, team 'away days'), it is a useful tool for building morale and relationships.

Finally, 'it is amazing what you can accomplish if you do not care who gets the credit' (President Harry S Truman, 1884–1972).

## Reference

9  Belbin RM. *Management Teams: why they succeed or fail*, 3rd edn. Routledge: New York, 2010.

## Further reading

Covey SR. *First Things First*. Simon & Schuster: London, 1994.
Katzenbach J. *The Wisdom of Teams: creating a high performance organisation*. McGraw Hill Publishing Co.: London, 2005.
Neil J. *What are Team Building Definitions?* ♫ www.wilderdom.com/teambuilding

# Leading an empowered organization

## What is leadership?

Leadership is about direction, and giving people a sense of purpose that inspires and motivates them to achieve. Leadership is also about a relationship between people—leaders and followers—that is built on shared values and trust.

Successfully leading an organization requires a complex balance between developing the people in it, managing its resources effectively, and ensuring that people sign up to and progress towards a shared vision. Most successful leaders have a well-defined sense of their own strengths and weaknesses. They do not try to be all things to all people. They are genuine and they develop a wide range of interpersonal skills.

## What skills make a leader?

According to Mary Bast, leadership skills are based on leadership behaviours.[10] She believes that skills alone do not make a leader, but style and behaviours do.

*Top five leadership behaviours*
- Integrity.
- Fairness.
- Prioritizing one's work.
- Being positive with oneself and others.
- Listening to people.

All empowered organizations try to build leadership capacity, as good leadership can promote substantial organizational performance. Poor leadership has the opposite effect, resulting in high turnover and absenteeism.

There are as many styles of leadership as there are leaders. The styles listed in Table 12.1 will be adapted to suit the organizational needs and existing style of the leader.[11]

## What successful leaders accomplish

Successful leaders lead positively charged or empowered organizations—they deliberately seek to increase the flow of positive emotions within an organization. Studies show that leaders who share positive emotions have staff who exhibit:[12]
- a more positive mood
- enhanced job satisfaction
- greater engagement and improved performance.

Finally, a great leader recognizes the input of others—large or small—to the organization's overall services. All input and effort should be acknowledged regularly. 'I praise loudly, I blame softly' (Catherine the Great, 1729–1796) is an excellent motto for aspiring leaders, even today.

**Table 12.1** Leadership styles in an empowered organization

| | |
|---|---|
| Visionary | They focus on long-term objectives and possibilities while developing a picture of the future. They encourage the teams around them to contribute to the vision, and they hold the values of the organization within the vision |
| Mentor | Healthy mentors are unconditionally caring leaders who derive satisfaction from encouraging the development of others. They support training throughout the organization |
| Democrat | They ensure that many voices are heard, placing a high value on inclusive communication. They use a range of mediums to convey their message, they are highly visible, and they 'walk the talk' |
| Diplomat | They bring cooperation to the work environment, and they enjoy building consensus and developing a shared sense of direction. They look for agreement and cohesion where possible |
| Innovator | They are vital to the health of an organization. They encourage risk taking, support new ideas, and are not bound by tradition. They enjoy challenging the status quo |

## References

10 Bast M. *Breakthroughs with the Enneagram*. ℘ www.internationalenneagram.org
11 Rath T and Clinton D. *How Full is Your Bucket?* Gallup Press: Princeton, NJ, 2005. See also ℘ www.bucketbook.com
12 Chapman A. *Ethical work and life learning, 1995–2014*. ℘ www.businessballs.com

# Managing effective teams

Nurses and other professional disciplines are increasingly expected to carry out managerial functions and have responsibility for a team. Managers require a diverse range of skills, and many feel threatened, especially in their first post. Often people with professional backgrounds have superb clinical skills but undeveloped managerial abilities. There are high costs if a team is not managed properly.

## The manager

Managers should have good leadership potential. However, the functions of a manager are more focused and specific than those of a leader. A manager will have:

- clearly stated aims and objectives for their team—delegated to them by the wider organization
- authority to manage and order the working day of the team
- responsibility to ensure that the team complies with the wider organizational framework and regulation.

## Management skills

In order to manage a team well, a manager will need to develop three groups of skills.

- *Communication*—clarity of vision and mission, clarity of expectation, fair, objective, and timely feedback, dissemination, and liaison with the wider organization.
- *Leadership*—inclusion of team members, appropriate delegation, respect, motivation, and inspiration.
- *Organization*—time and people management, capacity management, quality assurance, budget management, project planning, and performance management.

## Reasons why teams fail

- Lack of clearly defined aims and objectives for the team.
- Lack of a clear management mandate.
- Poor understanding of the corporate context in which the team operates.
- Poor internal relationships.
- Poor supporting systems, procedures, and processes (e.g. human resources, IT, clinical protocols).
- Poor communication—both within the team and in dissemination to and from the team within the wider organization.
- Poor levels of individual support, supervision, and development.
- Hindering behaviours and attitudes that are left unmanaged (e.g. gossip, boredom, lack of engagement, dominance of a few people, lack of listening).
- Actions often taken prematurely, prior to consultation, discussion, or planning.

## Reasons why teams succeed

- Clear goals and objectives that are clearly articulated and that are SMART (specific, measurable, achievable, realistic, and timed). These goals need to be established both for the team and for the individual in the annual appraisal process.
- Defined roles and functions that are clearly outlined in job descriptions and person specifications.
- Open and clear communication, including clarity of vision and expectation.
- Effective decision making.
- Balanced participation that recognizes the inputs of all team members, while acknowledging that the manager has the ultimate responsibility to decide upon the appropriate action required.
- Valuing of diversity.
- Management of conflict.
- Positive atmosphere.
- Effective systems and processes that provide a framework for effective functioning.

## Further reading

French WL, Bell CH and Zawacki RA. *Organisational Development and Transformation: managing effective change.* McGraw Hill Publishing Co.: London, 2004.

Makely S. *Professionalism in Health Care: a primer for career success,* 4th edn. Prentice Hall: Upper Saddle River, NJ, 2013.

# Clinical supervision

Clinical supervision, regardless of professional affiliation, should be a mechanism for protecting standards and public safety, while supporting the development of excellence in practice. It is basically a safe and confidential environment in which the dynamics of the working clinical world can be explored.

Not only are there a myriad of definitions, but there is also a proliferation of models. Some common features of clinical supervision are listed here.

- It has a number of aims, such as ensuring evidence-based practice, skills development, professional growth, and personal support for the practitioner.
- The process requires formal structures and procedures to make it safe and effective.
- It is an active process that requires equal input from the supervisee and the supervisor.

## Fundamentals of clinical supervision

At the very minimum, clinical supervision should help to:
- regulate standards
- develop professional function
- support the individual practitioner on a personal level.

Clinical supervision should not be confused with the following:
- *Appraisal*—this is a formal management process for the setting of job-specific aims and objectives. It is primarily guided by the needs of the organization (➜ Personal development and appraisal, p. 308).
- *Management supervision*—this is a formal process whereby a manager ensures that individuals who directly report to him or her are practising effectively, achieving specific goals and targets, and receiving regular feedback about their work-based performance (➜ Management supervision, p. 306).
- *Counselling*—this is a formal therapeutic activity (➜ Counselling, p. 56).
- *Mentoring*—this is an educational method whereby a student or learner is supported during a skills acquisition programme.
- *Caseload supervision*—this is a process that is primarily guided by the needs of the client or patient.

Clinical supervision differs from the activities listed in that it is primarily structured and governed by the needs of the supervisee as an autonomous practising individual, seeking guidance and structured enquiry into their practice. Clinical supervision is not something that is 'done to' anyone. It is not a mandatory process. It is an 'adult' process for practitioners exploring the dynamics of the clinical world in which they work.

Clinical supervision can be undertaken in a variety of ways. The most common formats are the one-to-one session or the group session. It is important that the clinical supervisor is not the manager of the supervisee and, where possible, the supervisee should have some say as to who their supervisor is. The supervisee needs to be satisfied that the supervisor has the appropriate skills and experience to assist them at whatever stage they are at in their professional life. All transactions should be entirely confidential, unless a breach of professional conduct is revealed during a clinical session. All issues regarding clinical supervision should be set down in a formal contract between the supervisor and the supervisee, with the basic ground rules being explained and agreed at the start of any supervision programme.

## Further reading

Bond M and Holland S. *Skills of Clinical Supervision for Nurses: a practical guide for supervisees, clinical supervisors and managers*. Open University Press: Maidenhead, 2011.

# Management supervision

This is an active management mechanism to ensure that directly managed employees are working to agreed targets and processes with appropriate outcomes. It is an opportunity for reflection and feedback. Unlike clinical supervision, it is a directly managed process, where the employee's work is the focus of the meeting. The agenda should be shared between the supervising manager and the employee, but this is not a self-directed meeting for the employee, and the outcomes of such meetings are very much focused on performance management.

Management supervision can be defined as a process whereby the supervisor meets with a member of staff to whom they have delegated key responsibilities. This supervisory meeting acts to coordinate, enhance, and evaluate the performance of the supervisee for whose work they are held accountable.

## Fundamentals of management supervision

Management supervision should:

- have an agreed plan that includes the workplace aims and objectives of the supervisee
- include the provision of guidance, direction, and feedback about performance, and the identification of training and development needs
- be integral to the annual performance appraisal process.

It is quite likely that the direct line manager will undertake management supervision. The supervisee will probably not have a choice in this matter. The process may feel challenging at times to all concerned, as the supervision will be based around the needs of the workplace and the ability of the supervisee to work in that environment.

Management supervision works best if the process is open, fair, and objective. Honest feedback is integral to the process. Some ground rules can be helpful:

- Rarely, poor performance issues may be discussed that require formal human resource processes to be put in place. The supervisee needs to be aware that this is a course of action open to the supervisor.
- All supervisors must adhere to the human resource policies of their organization, bearing in mind dignity at work, disciplinary, and grievance policies. Shouting, bullying, and aggression are unacceptable behaviours.
- The supervision should be facilitative and developmental, ensuring that the supervisee accomplishes their workplace objectives.
- The supervisor should provide an opportunity for the supervisee to discuss any ideas they may have about improving their performance in the workplace.
- All transactions should take place in an adult and respectful manner.

## Further reading

Reynolds A and Thornicroft G. *Managing Mental Health Services*. Open University Press: Buckingham, 1999.

# Personal development and appraisal

For an individual to perform well in the workplace, the organization needs to ensure that all employees:
- understand clearly what is expected of them with regard to workplace behaviour, aims, and objectives
- know the key mission of their organization
- are practically equipped to do the job that they are employed to do (e.g. they have access to a computer and a phone)
- are trained and developed appropriately so that they can deliver their objectives.

The appraisal is usually an annual meeting between the employee and their manager, where a focused discussion takes place. The purpose is to identify the forthcoming annual aims and objectives for the individual, together with a developmental plan that will ensure successful support. The appraisal is usually supplemented by quarterly progress meetings and management supervision.

## Fundamentals of appraisal

Appraisal is a formal developmental process of evaluation and structured discussion aimed at the personal, professional, and career development of the individual. Many organizations no longer combine this process with performance appraisal where the needs of the organization are at the forefront of the discussion.

At the very minimum, the appraisal should:
- actively include the individual in the organization—it should explain the key organizational mission and goals, and help the individual to understand how their role and department help the organization to succeed
- explain the aims, objectives, and targets that have been set for the appraiser and the specific department in which they work
- negotiate with the appraisee about what their own contribution to the departmental aims and objectives will be
- identify the training and development needs of the individual if they are to achieve their goals for the year
- contain objectives that are SMART (i.e. specific, measurable, achievable, realistic, and timed).

The appraisal should not:
- be regarded as an opportunity to suddenly cite the appraiser's concerns about the appraisee's performance—this meeting should contain no surprises
- be sprung upon the appraisee without adequate preparation time—the appraisee should have access to all the necessary paperwork well in advance
- be hurried or carried out in an inappropriate venue (e.g. phones should be diverted, and a 'do not disturb' sign should be hung on the door).

## The personal development plan

Relevant training and development opportunities should be identified that support the appraisee and help them to meet their aims and objectives. The opportunities identified should also consider the learning preferences of the appraisee. Training and development can be met in a variety of ways, including, for example:

- coaching or clinical supervision
- directed reading
- shadowing a colleague inside or outside the organization
- short visits or secondments to another department or situation
- joining a working party or task force
- joining a learning set
- attending conferences
- attending short courses
- attending longer courses or continuing with academic studies.

Note that health and safety training must be included as mandatory each year.

## Further reading

Baillie L and Black S. *Professional Values in Nursing*. CRC Press: Boca Raton, FL, 2014.

# The effective acute psychiatric ward

An effective acute psychiatric ward is one that:
- keeps patients as safe as possible
- accurately assesses the mental disorders and needs of each patient
- provides excellent care and treatment for mental and physical health problems
- assists, supports, and sometimes imposes self-care
- provides a respite location for patients, or by admitting a patient
- provides respite for their relatives or carers.

The fact that these are the functions of acute wards, and the standards by which their efficacy should be judged, is demonstrated by what staff say about their roles, and by the reasons for which patients are admitted.[13]

Running an effective ward is a whole-team function. Although much of the day-to-day burden is carried by mental health nurses, it requires input from psychiatrists, occupational therapists, support workers, and others. A ward cannot be effective unless the whole multidisciplinary team works together in partnership with shared ideals and values.

## Patient safety

Keeping patients safe means preventing them from harming themselves, others, and property. This sometimes requires coercion—for example, patients can be detained in hospital under the Mental Health Act 2007. Some argue that the best way to keep a patient safe is through the nurse–patient relationship, whereas others emphasize security policies and the use of containment, such as extra sedating medication or special observation. Both are required, but the most effective balance between them is subject to argument (see Table 12.2).

Table 12.2 Factors that affect ward safety

| Practice factors | Service factors |
|---|---|
| Risk assessment and predication | Ward design and ambience |
| De-escalation techniques | Social environment, case mix, forced cohabitation |
| Observation | |
| Physical intervention (use of restraint) | Amount of time staff spend with patients |
| Rapid tranquillization | Leadership, morale, use of bank and agency staff |

| System factors | Population factors |
|---|---|
| Clinical, service, and managerial systems that have an impact on ward safety | The ward will reflect the qualities of the community from which its patients are drawn |

## Assessment

For an accurate assessment, nurses require a thorough knowledge of psychopathology, and the ability to observe patient behaviour and record or communicate those observations in a clear, succinct, and objective manner. If a patient's needs go unnoticed or uncommunicated, their treatment may be compromised.

## Treatment

The provision of treatment by nurses should be undertaken with care and attention to detail. Treatment is usually consensual. However, due to the nature of mental disorder, it is occasionally legally coerced.

## Self-care

Acute mental illness affects a person's ability to care for him- or herself (e.g. to eat, drink, get enough sleep, stay clean, keep warm, and wear appropriate clothing). All of these deficits need to be identified and addressed by the effective nursing team working in partnership with patients.

## Reference

13 Bowers L, Clark N and Callaghan P. Multidisciplinary reflections on assessment for compulsory admission: the views of approved social workers, general practitioners, ambulance crews, community psychiatric nurses and psychiatrists. *British Journal of Social Work* 2003; **33**: 961–8.

## Further reading

The Schizophrenia Commission. *The Abandoned Illness: a report by the Schizophrenia Commission.* Rethink Mental Illness: London, 2012. ✍ www.rethink.org/media/514093/TSC_main_report_14_nov.pdf

# The effective community mental health team

## Introduction

The multidisciplinary team lies at the heart of modern health and social care. Collaboration between agencies and professional disciplines replaces divisions and demarcations, and improves the quality of service provision.

## Types of teams

- *Community mental health teams (CMHTs)*—these are generic teams that provide mental health care for the working-age population of a specific geographical area. Similar teams operate for older people (and are known as Older People CMHTs).
- *Assertive outreach teams (AOTs)*—these are specialist teams that provide assertive and intensive treatment for mentally ill people who frequently relapse and require inpatient treatment, and for those who are resistant to psychiatric treatment.
- *Home treatment or crisis teams*—these provide intensive care and support for people who would otherwise require admission to a psychiatric hospital, and for vulnerable people who have been discharged from hospital.
- *Early intervention teams*—these offer specialist treatment, information, and support to people who are experiencing their first psychotic illness.

Other specialist teams provide mental health services to members of black and minority ethnic (BME) communities, and to people who are homeless or who suffer from comorbid substance misuse problems.

## Effective teams

The effective care of severely mentally ill people requires a collaborative working relationship between psychiatrists, social workers, mental health nurses, and the service user. Optimal care requires the additional involvement of clinical psychologists, occupational therapists, support workers, and, increasingly, housing and welfare services, and those who work with refugees or asylum seekers. Where appropriate, constructive partnerships with primary care services and the family are essential.

Multidisciplinary health care teams that work effectively result in better patient outcomes, including reduced mortality, greater continuity of care, and consistent communication with patients and their families. They also develop shared knowledge and skills within the team.

Clear aims, policies, and procedures, and agreement on these, are crucial. Teams that have clear objectives, and higher levels of communication and member participation, operate more effectively. Greater integration and respect for team members is associated with new and innovative ways of delivering patient care, and improved mental well-being among staff.

Sufficient staff are required to provide a range of expertise and skills. However, large teams can become overwhelmed by communication and line management problems.

Effective CMHTs are associated with fewer suicides, greater continuity of care, shorter inpatient stays, less patient dissatisfaction, and lower costs.

# Collaborative care

'Collaborative care' is the term used to describe a systematic approach to supporting and organizing the management of people with high prevalence mental health problems such as depression and anxiety. It is characterized by close working relationships between those who use services with primary care generalists, such as GPs, non-statutory agencies, and housing and benefits offices, and specialist mental health professionals, mediated via case management principles.

Collaborative care has a very strong evidence base. A Cochrane Systematic Review in 2012 showed it consistently outperformed other systems with persistent beneficial results for people.

## Elements of collaborative care

Collaborative care has three elements:

- There are mechanisms to foster liaison between service users, primary care clinicians, and mental health specialists in relation to individual patient care. These include regular meetings between primary and secondary care specialists.
- A case manager supports and manages the needs of the service users through structured pharmacological and psychological interventions. Case managers deliver psychological support and provide holistic psychosocial biomedical intervention.
- There are mechanisms for collecting and sharing information on the progress of individual patients using shared information technology and primary care-based notes.

## Case management in collaborative care

Case management differs from traditional community mental health nursing practice in the following ways. Case managers:

- Hold large volumes of active cases, typically 100 or more.
- Use the telephone as the most common form of contact with patients.
- Undertake short contacts with patients, typically lasting no more than 10–20 minutes.
- Liaise primarily with primary care clinicians around the care of individual patients.
- Receive regular scheduled caseload supervision from mental health specialists.
- Proactively contact depressed patients identified by primary care clinicians, often trying many, many times to contact patients.
- Integrate medication support with protocolised evidence-based low-intensity psychological treatments such as problem solving, self-help CBT or behavioural activation.

## Further reading

Archer J, Bower P, Gilbody S et al. Collaborative care for depression and anxiety problems. *Cochrane Database of Systematic Reviews* 2012; **10**: CD006525. DOI: 10.1002/14651858.CD006525.pub2.
Richards DA, Hill JJ, Gask L et al. CADET: Clinical Effectiveness of Collaborative Care for Depression in UK Primary Care. A Cluster Randomised Controlled Trial. *British Medical Journal* 2013; **347**: f4913 doi: 10.1136/bmj.f4913.

# Promoting collaboration in primary mental health care

One in four people experience mental health problems of varying degrees of severity and complexity, and people may require different degrees of health and social support.

There is growing interest in examining effective ways in which people with mental health problems who are living in the community can be provided with and can access safe and responsive services. If the needs and aspirations of individuals are not adequately addressed, they will continue to face social exclusion. It is important that all agencies, including central government, the NHS, local government, the independent sector, and providers of housing and employment schemes are aware of the issues and prepared to take action. Current strategic government initiatives for the provision of quality care and support include access to evidence-based interventions, greater choice, recovery approaches, and a clear focus on human rights.[14,15]

⧖ Mental health and well-being in the global context, p. 4.
⧖ Strategic visions for mental health nursing, p. 4.

## Reasons why people with mental health problems do not engage with mental health services
- Upbringing, life experiences, or attitudes.
- Feeling let down in the past.
- Stigma and discrimination.
- Negative staff attitudes (e.g. racism or homophobia).
- Staff lacking the necessary skills.
- The use of purely biomedical approaches.
- Lack of family or carer support.
- Lack of knowledge or information.

Mental health services may not be able to engage effectively with individuals, families, and carers due to factors such as the need to prioritize care, staff competencies, lack of time, and lack of resources.

## The needs of service users
In a paper published by the Centre for Mental Health in 2012,[16] it is reported that when service users were asked what they needed from services, their responses included the following:
- engagement and someone to talk to
- a range of treatments and care, including crisis intervention
- the availability of an identified responsible person, 24 hours a day
- a risk management approach that maximizes the safety of the service user and the public
- consideration of social factors as well as mental and medical problems
- supported access to mainstream services
- daytime activity—to provide occupation, opportunity, and purpose
- help with managing finances and benefits
- suitable accommodation
- living and working skills.

## Recommendations for delivering effective and responsive health and social care

A government workforce team made the following recommendations for delivering effective health and social care that is responsive to the needs of people with mental health problems:[17]

- skilled staff, including training and supervision of those staff
- talking therapies
- new roles (e.g. graduate mental health workers, gateway workers)
- needs-led services
- staff who are able to work in informal settings
- effective joint working for statutory and non-statutory sectors
- a shared vision and common agenda
- development of positive staff attitudes in primary care
- a focus on psychosocial interventions
- support for families and carers
- the development of mental health awareness in schools, colleges, and the workplace
- assertive outreach, and a caseload ceiling of ten service users
- more prison in-reach staff
- community development workers for BME communities
- outreach teams for service users with personality disorder.

The overall aim is to develop a workforce with the competencies to provide person-centred, socially inclusive, and recovery-focused services in a multidisciplinary setting. To foster engagement, the service user and their carers should be fully involved in decision making, given informed choices, and treated with dignity and respect.

## References

14 Department of Health. *No Health Without Mental Health: a cross-government mental health outcomes strategy for people of all ages*. Department of Health: London, 2011.

15 Department of Health. *Talking Therapies: a four-year plan of action*. Department of Health: London, 2011.

16 Centre for Mental Health. *Recovery, Public Mental Health and Wellbeing*. Centre for Mental Health: London, 2012.

17 National Institute for Mental Health (England) and Mental Health Care Group Workforce Team. *Mental Health Workforce Strategy*. Department of Health: London, 2004.

# Multi-agency working

Mental health nursing takes place in the context of work with other agencies that are also involved in the care of service users. In this section we shall consider how mental health nurses can work effectively with other agencies.

## Advantages of multi-agency working

- More efficient use of staff.
- Effective service provision.
- A more satisfying work environment.
- More effective achievement of objectives.
- Seamless delivery of care.
- Less medicalization of mental health problems.
- Provision of a medium for mental health awareness.
- Promotion of an inclusive form of mental health care.

## Working effectively with other agencies

In order to work effectively with other agencies, the mental health nurse needs to:

- be capable of explaining their role and the parameters within which they work
- be capable of communicating with other agencies
- understand the role and boundaries of other agencies
- be capable of engaging service users in collaborative working across agencies by empowering and informing them (e.g. explaining the role of other agencies, such as children and families social services)
- recognize the part that significant others play in supporting the service user.

## Multi-agency teams

Mental health nurses work with other agencies in the following teams:

- CMHTs
- AOTs
- home treatment or crisis teams
- early intervention teams
- other specialist teams (e.g. those that provide mental health services to members of BME communities, or to people who are homeless or who have comorbid substance misuse problems).

It is also important to acknowledge the inter-agency capacity within the role of the acute inpatient nurse, who will have to liaise and negotiate with other agencies such as the police, the Mental Health Act Commission, and independent advocacy services, as well as all of the statutory authorities, such as approved social workers.

## Health and social care organizations

Mental health nurses may work with the following health and social care organizations:

- social services
- the Department for Work and Pensions
- groups involved in mental health care and support (e.g. Mind, SANE, Rethink, Mental Health Foundation)
- the Mental Health Act Commission
- the Care Quality Commission
- local authority housing departments and housing associations.

They may also work with cultural diversity agencies, such as:

- Jewish Care
- the Chinese Mental Health Association.

# Working with advocacy services

Advocacy refers to the process of pleading the cause of and acting on behalf of another person, in order to secure the services that they need and the rights to which they are entitled. Advocates are independent of service providers, and represent the interests of their advocacy partner as if they were their own.

Advocacy takes many shapes and forms, and provides both challenges and opportunities for nurses.

### Self-advocacy

Self-advocacy involves individuals speaking out for themselves, and acting on their own behalf. They might be supported by groups such as the following:

- *Self-help groups*—for people with particular diagnoses, or similar experiences (e.g. sexual abuse survivors, or people from minority ethnic communities).
- *Survivor groups*—campaigning independently, rather than working alongside service providers.
- *Advocacy projects and patients' councils*—working in a locality to support service users on hospital wards or in the community.
- *Service user forums*—local groups seeking changes, who participate in the planning, research, and evaluation of local mental health services, and provide training for mental health workers.

Some of these groups may not fall neatly into one category, but may have several functions.

### Group advocacy

Group advocacy involves the empowerment of groups to speak and be heard on specific issues (e.g. a patients' council, or a user group for a particular service). As well as being valuable sources of information and mutual support, these groups are able to give their opinions on services, and lobby for new services or improvements to existing services. Advocacy groups can also decide to set up and run their own services, which may range, for example, from social clubs to crisis houses.

### Peer advocacy

This involves an individual being given the support of an advocate who has themselves used, or is using, mental health services.

### Legal advocacy

Legal advocacy is representation by legally qualified advocates, who are usually solicitors. Some will specialize in service users detained under the Mental Health Act 2007.

### Citizen advocacy

This is a long-term, one-to-one partnership between a service user and an advocate who is a member of the public, usually as part of a scheme coordinated by an organization or service.

## Formal or professional advocacy

This refers to advocacy schemes that are staffed by paid professionals. They may be managed by large voluntary organizations. They sometimes adopt a so-called 'expert' model of advocacy, which involves giving advice, prioritizing options, counselling, and mediation services.

## Nurses working with advocacy services

When working with advocacy services, nurses should:
- adhere to any working agreements with the advocacy service
- respect the independence and principles of the advocacy service
- be aware of confidentiality issues (who tells whom what)
- involve advocates in any health care meetings that the nurse holds with his or her patients
- adhere to their employer's information-sharing policy.

## Further reading

UK Advocacy Network (UKAN) website. ℘ www.u-kan.co.uk

UK Advocacy Network (UKAN). *Advocacy: a code of practice*. UKAN: Sheffield, 1994.

UK Advocacy Network (UKAN). *A Clear Voice, A Clear Vision: the advocacy reader*. UKAN: Sheffield, 2001.

UK Advocacy Network (UKAN). *Advocacy Today and Tomorrow: the UK Advocacy Network training tool*. UKAN: Sheffield, 2004.

# Evidence-based mental health nursing

**Patrick Callaghan**

# Introduction to evidence-based practice

Evidence-based practice is defined by Sackett and colleagues[1] as 'the integration of best research evidence with clinical experience and values.'

## What is evidence?

Evidence includes the following:
- the results of well-designed research studies, irrespective of the methodology
- data from studies such as randomized controlled trials (RCTs) that test effectiveness and efficacy
- advice from experts endorsed by respected authorities
- clinical assessments of patients based on information gathered
- beliefs and values of practitioners
- patients' preferences and choices.

## Assessing the quality of evidence

Asking the following questions can help to establish the quality of evidence:
- Is this the best type of research method to answer this question?
- Is the research of adequate quality?
- What is the size of the beneficial effect and of the adverse effect?
- Is it possible to generalize the findings of the research to the whole population from which the sample was drawn?
- How transferable might the results be to other populations?
- Are the results applicable to the 'local' population?
- Are the results applicable to this patient or service user?

## The components of evidence-based practice

- The success or harm of all interventions.
- Clinical guidelines.
- Patient and public choice.
- Information on epidemiology.
- Evidence-based purchasing that reflects audit outcomes and performance measures.
- Health service management.
- Organizational audit.
- Financial audit and guidelines.
- Education and training.
- Curricula based on best possible and available evidence.

## Skills required by the evidence-based mental health nurse

These skills include an ability to:
- define criteria such as effectiveness, safety, and acceptability
- find articles on the effectiveness, safety, and acceptability of a new test or treatment
- assess the quality of evidence
- assess whether the findings of the research can be generalized to the whole population from which the sample was drawn
- assess whether the findings of the research are applicable to the 'local' population.

## Critique of evidence-based practice
- The premise that health care should be based on the best available evidence is sound.
- Evidence-based practice is an authoritarian gesture with the purpose of bringing about conformity and compliance with questionable dogma.
- At what point is enough evidence gathered to justify a clinical decision?
- The integration of clinical acumen with current best evidence will improve competence and caring in health professionals.
- Health problems are not neatly resolved by recourse to research trials and hierarchies of evidence.
- Questions relating to the care of patients are not all answered by science.
- Health care is at the interface of many disciplines, not just epidemiology, as evidence-based practice seems to imply.
- The role of other types of evidence—such as that derived from qualitative research—has not been clearly delineated in evidence-based practice.

## Best value: a complement to evidence-based practice?
Best value is a means of achieving improvements in social care that also has value for improving health care alongside evidence-based practice.

*Factors that are necessary to achieve best value in nursing*
- Ownership of problems and willingness to change.
- A sustained focus on what matters.
- The capacity and systems to deliver performance and improvement.
- Integration of best value principles into all activities.

*Principles for modernizing care using a best value approach*
- Organizing services around people.
- Empowering people and supporting them to live their lives in the way that they choose.
- A step change approach to improving services, so that service users experience tangible changes.
- Recognizing and responding to the needs of carers.
- Delivering services in a seamless way.
- Ensuring that services are sensitive to the needs of under-represented and minority populations.
- Developing a confident and well-supported workforce.

## Evidence-based health: a movement in crisis?
A recently published paper by Greenhalgh and colleagues[2] analyses progress in evidence-based medicine in the past 20 years and reflects upon its current state. The key points can be summarized as follows:
- The evidence-based quality mark has been misappropriated by vested interests.
- The volume of evidence has become unmanageable.
- Statistically significant benefits may be marginal in practice.
- Inflexible rules and technology-driven changes are often management driven, rather than being driven by patient needs.
- Evidence-based guidelines often map poorly to complexity problems.

### Evidence-based health: a new focus

Real evidence-based health:[2]
- prioritizes ethical care of patients
- presents evidence in a format that is easy for staff and patients to understand
- is characterized by expert judgement
- involves shared decision making with patients
- emphasizes robust clinician–patient relationships and the human aspects of care
- uses these principles in all areas of health, including public health.

### Actions to deliver real evidence-based health

- Patients must demand better evidence, which is better presented, better explained, and applied personally.
- Staff training must focus on honing clinical judgement and shared decision-making skills.
- Producers of evidence summaries must account fully for who will use them.
- Publishers should ensure that studies address usability as well as methodological concerns.
- Policy makers should avoid use of evidence by vested interests.
- Funders must shape the production, synthesis, and dissemination of high-quality evidence.
- The research agenda must be broader and more interdisciplinary.

### References

1 Sackett DL et al. *Evidence-Based Medicine: how to practice and teach EBM.* Churchill Livingstone: New York, 2000. p. 71.
2 Greenhalgh T, Howick J and Maskrey N. Evidence-based medicine: a movement in crisis? *British Medical Journal* 2014; **348**: g3725. ℅ www.bmj.com/content/348/bmj.g3725

### Further reading

Gray JAM. *Evidence-Based Health Care and Public Health*, 3rd edn. Churchill-Livingstone: London, 2009.
Social Services Inspectorate and Audit Commission. *Getting the Best from Best Value: the experience of applying best value in social care.* Department of Health: London, 2002.

# Evaluating published evidence

The term 'evaluate' means to judge the worth or value of something. Evaluation requires a balanced critique during which the strengths and weaknesses of the published paper are identified. Most research textbooks have a section on how to evaluate a published paper. The revised CONSORT statement[3] offers useful guidance on critiquing RCTs. An excellent example is found in Polit and Beck,[4] and another helpful example is Benton and Cormack.[5] In addition, the Critical Appraisal Skills Programme (CASP) website[6] has 10 different checklists for critiquing 10 different types of research reports, and is an indispensable source of useful information for critiquing research (see Table 13.1).

## General tips on evaluating published research

- Be as objective as possible.
- Do not insult the author(s) or question their competence.
- Be reasonable in your critique.
- Give specific examples of the strengths and limitations of the paper.
- Be sensitive when making negative statements; put yourself in the authors' shoes.
- Try to justify your criticisms.
- Suggest alternatives.

**Table 13.1** Checklists and tools to help to evaluate published studies[3]

| Research design | Checklist and source |
| --- | --- |
| Randomized controlled trial (RCT) | CONSORT Statement<br>🔊 www.consort-statement.org |
| Clustered RCT | CONSORT Plus<br>🔊 www.consort-statement.org/extensions |
| Non-randomized evaluations | TREND<br>🔊 www.cdc.gov/trendstatement |
| Observational studies in epidemiology | STROBE Statement<br>🔊 www.strobe-statement.org |
| Studies that test diagnostic accuracy | STARD Statement<br>🔊 www.stard-statement.org |
| Meta-analysis and systematic reviews | PRISMA Statement<br>🔊 www.prisma-statement.org |
| Evaluating ethical probity of studies | ASSERT Statement<br>🔊 www.assert-statement.org/explanatorydocument.html |

## The evaluation process

Most research reports are written using a particular structure, with subsections describing each part of the research undertaken. You can use this structure to form your evaluation. In particular, your evaluation may focus on the following:

- researchers' qualifications
- title
- abstract
- introduction
- background and literature review
- theoretical and conceptual framework
- research aims, questions, and hypotheses (if any)
- definition of key terms
- research design
- population and sample
- data collection methods
- data collection instruments (if any)
- data analysis
- discussion of findings
- conclusions
- implications
- recommendations
- overall impression.

## General tips on evaluating published research-based evidence[7]

- Abstract:
  - Does the abstract provide a clear summary of the research paper, including the research question and the methods applied?
  - Are the key findings and the conclusions stated?
- Research question:
  - Does the research paper identify a research question or hypothesis?
  - Is that question or hypothesis followed through into the conclusion?
  - Were the chosen methods appropriate to the question at hand?
- Literature review:
  - Is the literature review comprehensive and up to date?
  - Are any gaps in the literature identified?
  - Does the literature review support the case for further research?
- Methodology:
  - Does the research paper indicate the research approach that it is adopting?
  - How relevant is the methodological framing of the research?
  - Are the best methods applied to answer the research question?
- Sample:
  - Is the sample size included?
  - Is the sample size appropriate to the aims of the research?
  - Are the characteristics of the sample described?
  - Is the response rate stated?

- Data collection:
  - What method was used to collect the data?
  - How valid and reliable are the methods?
- Data analysis:
  - Does the research paper state how the data were analysed?
  - Were these methods appropriate?
- Discussion and conclusion:
  - Does the paper provide a balanced account or discussion of the findings?
  - Were the limitations of the research indicated?
  - Do the conclusions match the findings?
  - Were the recommendations reasonable or credible?

## Key points
- It is important how you read, not just what you read.
- Being critical is a process, not an attitude.
- Use published criteria to help you to review research papers.

## References
3 Moher D et al. CONSORT 2010 explanation and elaboration: updated guidelines for reporting parallel group randomised trials. *British Medical Journal* 2010; **340**: c869.
4 Polit DF and Beck CT. *Essentials of Nursing Research: appraising evidence for nursing practice*, 8th edn. Lippincott Williams & Wilkins: Philadelphia, PA, 2013.
5 Benton DC and Cormack DFS. Reviewing and evaluating the literature. In: DFS Cormack (ed.) *The Research Process in Nursing*, 4th edn. Blackwell Science: Oxford, 2000. pp. 69–84.
6 Critical Appraisal Skills Programme (CASP) website. ℘ www.casp-uk.net
7 Callaghan P and Crawford P. Evidence-based mental health nursing practice. In: P Callaghan, J Playle and L Cooper (eds) *Mental Health Nursing Skills*. Oxford University Press: Oxford, 2006. pp. 33–43.

# Clinical governance

Clinical governance is central to the UK Government's drive for quality improvements in the NHS. It is the framework for delivering health services, and it is a method of helping services to achieve the standards set out in the various National Service Frameworks.

Clinical governance provides the means to ensure local delivery of excellent care using the evidence provided by the National Institute for Health and Care Excellence (NICE). The Care Quality Commission (CQC) monitors services to make sure that the best available evidence is being used.

## What is clinical governance?

Clinical governance is the method used by NHS organizations to deliver care and to account for the quality of that care.

## Features of clinical governance

- *Effective leadership*—where the vision, values, and methods of clinical governance are communicated to all staff.
- *Planning for quality*—a plan to develop quality services is established based on an objective assessment of the needs and views of service users, and exposure to risk. It identifies regulatory requirements, staff capabilities, unmet training needs, and an appreciation of how performance compares with best practice and similar services.
- *Being truly service user-centred*—this involves being clear about how feedback from service users contributes to service planning and delivery.
- *Information, analysis, and insight*—this means having excellent systems for selecting, managing, and using information.
- *Good service design*—this involves reflecting upon how services are designed, and changing services so that they are better designed to meet service users' needs if necessary.
- *Demonstrating success*—measures of quality and effectiveness are developed and used to demonstrate success.

## Does clinical governance lead to better care?[8,9]

- Clinical governance has led to greater and more explicit accountability.
- It has also led to more open, transparent, and collaborative ways of working.
- The implementation of clinical governance is patchy across trusts.
- Trusts view clinical governance as having led to achievements in the structure and process of care delivery.
- The parts of clinical governance that meet statutory requirements without necessarily meeting the needs of patients are the most robust of all its components.

There is no direct evidence that improvements linked to clinical governance are directly improving patient care. There may be indirect improvements, as seen in the CQC's Performance Ratings of Trusts, and in evidence from the National Patient Experience Surveys. However:

- Errors and inconsistencies were found in Trust documentation.
- Clinical governance was poorly understood in practice.
- Corporate goals were not shared.
- The impact of clinical governance in improving quality was inconsistent in practice.

## References

8 National Audit Office. *Achieving Improvements Through Clinical Governance*. National Audit Office: London, 2003.
9 Staniland K. A sociological and ethnographic study of clinical governance in one NHS Hospital Trust. *Clinical Governance: an International Journal* 2009; **14**: 271–80.

## Further reading

McSherry R and Pearce P. *Clinical Governance: a guide to implementation for healthcare professionals*. Wiley-Blackwell: London, 2011.

# Clinical audit

Clinical audit is a system designed to ensure that health care is delivered in line with agreed standards so that health service users know how well their services are doing and how they could be improved. Clinical audit is central to clinical governance. The National Clinical Audit and Patient Outcomes Programme (NCAPOP)[10] commissions and manages 30 national audits on behalf of the NHS in England.

### Areas covered by the NCAPOP

These include:
- cancer
- acute care
- mental health
- long-term conditions
- older people
- heart conditions
- women's and children's health.

### Clinical Outcome Review Programmes (CORP)

The CORP[11] have replaced the national confidential enquiries programme, and are designed to assess the quality of health care and stimulate improvements in key areas of work through the Healthcare Quality Improvement Partnership (HQIP). The current focus is on:
- medicine and surgery
- mental health
- child health
- maternal, newborn, and infant health
- asthma
- child head injuries.

### Features of effective clinical audit

- It should be part of a structured programme.
- Topics chosen for audit should be high risk, high volume, or high cost.
- Service should be part of the audit process.
- The audit should be multidisciplinary in nature.
- It should include assessment of the process and outcome of care.
- Standards should be derived from good-quality guidelines.
- The sample size chosen should be sufficient to produce credible outcomes.
- Managers should be directly involved in audit and any action plans arising from it.
- Action plans should address barriers to change, and identify those responsible for service improvement.
- Re-audit should be applied to ascertain whether improvements in care are a result of clinical audit.
- Systems, structures, and specific mechanisms should be made available to monitor service improvements once the audit cycle is complete.
- Each audit should have a local lead.

## The link between clinical audit and service improvement

Using clinical audit, service providers can examine whether:

- what ought to be happening is happening
- current practice meets required standards
- current practice follows published guidelines
- clinical practice is applying the knowledge that has been gained through research
- current evidence is being applied in a given situation.

There is no direct evidence that clinical audit leads directly to improvements in patient care. There may be indirect improvements as evidenced by the CQC's Performance Ratings of Trusts and evidence from the National Patient Experience Surveys. In the evaluation of clinical governance published by the National Audit Office in 2003,[12] clinical audit was perceived as extremely effective by one trust, as very effective by 20 trusts, and as fairly effective by 61 trusts, whereas it was perceived as not very effective by 17 trusts, and not at all effective by 1 trust.

## References

10  Healthcare Quality Improvement Partnership (HQIP). *National Clinical Audit Programme.* ℘ www.hqip.org.uk/national-clinical-audits-managed-by-hqip

11  Healthcare Quality Improvement Partnership (HQIP). *Clinical Outcome Review Programmes.* ℘ www.hqip.org.uk/clinical-outcome-review-programmes-2/

12  National Audit Office. *Achieving Improvements through Clinical Governance: a progress report on implementation by NHS trusts.* National Audit Office: London, 2003.

## Further reading

McSherry R and Pearce P. *Clinical Governance: a guide to implementation for healthcare professionals.* Wiley-Blackwell: London, 2011.

Staniland K. A sociological and ethnographic study of clinical governance in one NHS Hospital Trust. *Clinical Governance: an International Journal* 2009; **14**: 271–80.

# Clinical guidelines

Clinical guidelines are systematically developed statements that assist clinicians and patients in making decisions about appropriate treatment for specific conditions. The use of clinical guidelines is now widespread in many countries, and the evidence suggests that they do improve clinical practice, although the size of improvements varies greatly. Clinical guidelines are similar in many respects to care pathways, and sometimes these terms are used synonymously (see Table 13.2).

## The purpose of clinical guidelines
- They assist clinical decision making by patients and practitioners.
- They educate individuals and groups.
- They assess and ensure the quality of care.
- They guide the allocation of resources.
- They reduce the risk of legal liability for negligent care.

## Suitable areas for development of clinical guidelines
- Where there is excessive morbidity, disability, or mortality.
- Where treatment offers significant potential to reduce morbidity, disability, or mortality.
- Where there is wide variation in clinical practice.
- Where the services involved are resource intensive—either high volume and low cost, or low volume and high cost.
- Where there are many boundary issues involved, sometimes cutting across primary, secondary, and community care, and sometimes across different professional bodies.

**Table 13.2** Factors that influence the effectiveness of clinical guidelines

| Relative probability of being effective | Development strategy | Dissemination strategy | Implementation strategy |
|---|---|---|---|
| High | Internal group | Specific educational intervention | Patient-specific reminder at time of consultation or treatment |
| Above average | Intermediate group | Continuing professional development | Patient-specific feedback |
| Below average | Local external group | Mailing to targeted groups | General feedback |
| Low | National external group | Publication in professional journal | General reminder of guideline |

## Benefits and drawbacks of clinical guidelines

*Benefits*
- Provision of holistic care.
- Greater interprofessional collaboration.
- Provision of a seamless package of care.
- Failure to achieve outcomes is quickly identified, as expected outcomes at different stages are specified.
- Unmet needs can be identified.
- Treatment variation should be reduced.
- Closer involvement of service users.
- Care can be properly audited.
- The opportunity for effective and efficient care is maximized.
- Empowerment of service users.

*Drawbacks*
- They may be rejected by clinicians because of constraints.
- They were initially developed in the USA to control costs.
- They may restrict the freedom of clinicians.
- Deviations from guidelines may be time consuming and costly.
- They assume that robust evidence exists—where it does not, there may not be agreement on the most appropriate treatment.

## Procedure for developing clinical guidelines
- Select a suitable topic.
- Map the current process.
- Develop a guideline.
- Consult with service providers and users.
- Seek a consensus.
- Implement the guideline.
- Evaluate the guideline.
- Redesign the guideline if necessary.

## Factors linked to the success of clinical guidelines (National Institute of Clinical Studies (NICS), Australia[13])
- The dissemination strategies used.
- The implementation strategies used.
- The methods used to evaluate the guidelines.
- The methods used to update the guidelines.
- The clinical setting.

## The effect of clinical guidelines on practice: the evidence
Multifaceted interventions have been shown to result in mild to moderate improvements in care.[14]

Guidelines appear to change the processes and outcomes of care, with seven out of nine studies reporting improvements in infection rates and symptom relief.[15]

## References

13  National Institute of Clinical Studies (NICS), Australia. *Do Guidelines Make a Difference to Health Care Outcomes?* ℘ www.nhmrc.gov.au/_files_nhmrc/file/nics/material_resources/Do%20guidelines%20make%20a%20difference%20to%20health%20care%20outcomes.pdf
14  Grimshaw JM et al. Effectiveness and efficiency of guideline dissemination and implementation strategies. *Health Technology Assessment* 2004; **8**: 1–72.
15  Thomas L et al. Guidelines in professions allied to medicine. *Cochrane Database of Systematic Reviews* 2000; **2**: CD000349.

## Further reading

National Institute of Health and Care Excellence (NICE). *The Guideline Development Process: an overview for stakeholders, the public and the NHS*, 3rd edn. NICE: London, 2007.

# The National Institute for Health and Care Excellence (NICE)[16]

NICE is responsible for providing national guidance on the promotion of good health and the prevention and treatment of ill health. It aims to combine knowledge and guidance on how to promote health and treat ill health. Healthcare Improvement Scotland issues alerts and and advises NHS Scotland on the applicability of NICE guidance in Scotland. The Department of Health, Social Services and Public Safety in Northern Ireland uses NICE guidance, guidance from the Social Care Institute for Excellence (SCIE), its own guidance, and Clinical Resource Efficiency Support Team (CREST) guidance. NICE also provides public health guidance.

## Guidance produced by NICE

NICE produces three main types of guidance on a range of health problems and issues:

- *Technology appraisals*—guidance on the use of new and existing medicines and treatments within the NHS in England and Wales.
- *Clinical guidelines*—guidance on the appropriate treatment and care of people with specific diseases and conditions within the NHS in England and Wales.
- *Interventional procedures*—guidance on whether interventional procedures used for diagnosis or treatment are safe enough and work well enough for routine use in England, Wales, and Scotland.

## The role of NICE in evidence-based health care

Within the NHS, clinical governance is the means of ensuring local delivery of excellent care based on evidence, some of which is provided by NICE. The CQC monitors services to make sure that the best available evidence is being used.

→ Assessing the quality of health services: the role of the Care Quality Commission, p. 340.

## Reference

16  National Institute for Health and Care Excellence (NICE) website. ℘ www.nice.org.uk

## Assessing the quality of health services: the role of the Care Quality Commission

### Introduction

The Care Quality Commission (CQC) is the independent regulator for monitoring the quality of health care in England (see Table 13.3). The Healthcare Improvement Scotland and Care and Social Services Inspectorate Wales (CSSIW) play a similar role in focusing upon being assured that services are person-centred, safe and effective and those receiving care are treated with respect, compassion and dignity. The CQC's role is to check whether hospitals, care homes, GPs, dentists, and services provided in people's homes meet national standards.

**Table 13.3** Care Quality Commission standards

| National standards | Essential standards: outcomes that the CQC expects all people using services to receive | Other standards: criteria for assessing day-to-day management of services |
|---|---|---|
| Service users should expect to be respected, involved in their care, supported, and told what is happening at every stage | Respecting and involving people who use services | Fees |
| | Consent to care and treatment | Statement of purpose |
| | | Notification of the death of a service user |
| Service users should expect to receive care, treatment, and support that meets their needs | Care and welfare of people who use services | Notification of the death or unauthorized absence of a person who is detained or liable to be detained under the Mental Health Act 2007 |
| | Meeting nutritional needs | |
| Care should be safe | Cooperating with other providers | |
| Service users should expect to be cared for by staff with the right skills to do their jobs properly | Safeguarding service users from abuse | Notification of other incidents |
| | Cleanliness and infection control | Requirements where the service provider is an individual or partnership |
| | Management of medicines | |
| Service users should expect their care provider to routinely check the quality of their services | Safety and suitability of premises | Requirements where the service provider is a body other than a partnership |
| | Safety, availability, and suitability of equipment | |
| | Requirements relating to workers | Requirements relating to registered managers |
| | Assessing and monitoring the quality of service provision | Registered person: training |
| | Complaints | Financial position |
| | Records | Notifications: notice of absence |
| | | Notifications: notice of changes |

## Key roles of the CQC
- To *regulate* all health and social care provision.
- To *check* all services.
- To *inspect* all services to ensure that they comply with agreed standards.

## Inspection and regulation by the CQC
- Most services are inspected at least once each year.
- Dental services are inspected at least every 2 years.
- Inspectors are accompanied by subject experts or experts by experience.
- There are three types of inspection visits:
  - *scheduled*—inspections carried out in a rolling programme but not notified to the provider
  - *themed*—visits to a particular type of service
  - *responsive*—visits where there are concerns raised about a provider's services.
- Following an inspection a provider is judged to be either compliant or non-compliant with the standards.
- Reports of all inspections are published on the CQC website.[17]
- Information of relevance to the CQC in making judgements is gathered through a Quality and Risk Profile (QRP), notifications from providers, and provider compliance assessments in which providers can assess their own quality assurance.

**Reference**
17 Care Quality Commission (CQC) website. ℘ www.cqc.org.uk

# Disseminating and implementing evidence to improve practice

The overall aim of systematic reviews and clinical guidelines is to improve the quality of health care, and in the long term to improve health outcomes. However, this will only happen if the evidence generated by reviews is incorporated into policy and practice. Clinical guidelines are one way of getting evidence into practice.

Different methods of dissemination and implementation that have been shown to be effective in incorporating evidence into practice can be summarized as follows:

- *Dissemination*—the process whereby target groups become aware of, receive, accept, and utilize information.
- *Diffusion*—a passive process whereby information is spread to an audience.
- *Implementation*—activities aimed at improving the compliance of the target group with the recommendations about changes in clinical practice and health policy.

## Evidence-based methods of effective dissemination and implementation

- Academic detailing—providing lectures.[18]
- Opinion leaders—people who are regarded as influential and credible.
- Audit and feedback.
- Reminder systems.
- Patient-mediated interventions.

## Consistently effective interventions

- Educational outreach visits.
- Reminders.
- Multifaceted interventions (e.g. two or more of audit and feedback reminders, local consensus processes, and marketing).
- Interactive educational meetings.

## Interventions of variable effectiveness

- Audit and feedback.
- Local opinion leaders.
- Local consensus processes.
- Patient-mediated interventions.

## Interventions that have little or no effect

- Educational materials.
- Didactic educational meetings.

**Putting evidence into practice: a report from 15 projects funded by the London Regional Office of the NHS ME**

*Factors related to likelihood of success*
- Sufficient resources (e.g. time. money, and skills).
- Proposed change offers benefits to front-line staff.
- Enough of the right people are on board early enough.
- Interactive approach linking research clearly to practice.

*Key lessons of the project*
- Expect it to take several years.
- Successful implementation requires pragmatism and flexibility.
- Start small and build incrementally.
- Use what is already there.
- Target enthusiasts first.

*Outcomes of the project*
- Better relationships.
- Improved knowledge, systems, and skills.
- Change in practice.
- Improved patient care.

## Effective innovations in service delivery organizations

These include:
- innovations that have a clear advantage to those who are using them[19]
- innovations that are compatible with the values and needs of those who are using them
- simple innovations
- innovations that have been trialled through piloting
- clearly visible innovations
- innovations that can be refined by end users to suit their situation
- low-risk innovations (risky innovations are less likely to be adopted)
- innovations that end users feel will improve their performance.

## References

18 Bero LA et al. Closing the gap between research and practice: an overview of systematic reviews of interventions to promote the implementation of research findings. *British Medical Journal* 1998; **317**: 465–8.

19 Greenhalgh T et al. Diffusion of innovations in service organisations: systematic review and recommendations. *The Milbank Quarterly* 2004; **82**: 581–629.

## Further reading

Wye L and McClenahan J. *Getting Better with Evidence: experiences of putting evidence into practice.* The King's Fund: London, 2000.

# Systematic reviews

A systematic review is a review of the evidence on a clearly formulated question. It uses systematic and explicit methods to identify, select, and critically appraise relevant primary research and to extract and analyse data from the studies that are included in the review. Statistical methods (meta-analysis) may or may not be used.

## Strengths of systematic reviews

- They give comprehensive coverage—they may include studies using various research methods.
- Large amounts of information can be summarized concisely.
- Data from previous studies can be re-analysed, to present a composite picture.
- They are a useful aid to practitioners' pursuit of evidence-based health care.
- They can assist in the formation of effective social and health policy.
- They provide information on the effectiveness of an intervention.
- They reduce the need for guesswork on the part of readers.

## Weaknesses of systematic reviews

- There may be subjectivity in the inclusion, analysis, and reporting of data, because ultimately it is the reviewers who decide what is included.
- Coverage of the topic is restricted by the specific inclusion criteria.
- The effects of an intervention could be explained by many variables, not just the ones that are reported.
- Data from the studies may not be homogeneous.
- The studies may be combined inappropriately— that is, studies using different methods or different participants may be analysed together.

## Stages of the systematic review process

- Identification of the need for a review.
- Background research and problem specification.
- Drawing up the requirements for the review protocol.
- Literature searching and retrieval.
- Assessment of studies for inclusion.
- Assessment of the validity of studies.
- Data extraction.
- Data synthesis.
- Report writing.

## Methods of identifying evidence for inclusion in systematic reviews

- Database searching.
- Hand searching.
- Searching reference lists of identified studies.
- Contacting researchers in the field.
- Finding unpublished literature.

## Evaluating the quality of systematic reviews

The PRISMA checklist is designed to enable readers to evaluate the quality of systematic reviews (PRISMA can be accessed via ✍ www.prisma-statement.org). The checklist contains 14 items that a well-designed systematic review should include. In addition to using PRISMA, the following questions may help you to evaluate a systematic review:

- Does the review answer a well-defined question?
- Has there been a substantial effort to search for all of the available literature (including unpublished literature)?
- Are the inclusion and exclusion criteria reported and appropriate?
- Is the validity of all of the included studies adequately addressed?
- Are the individual studies presented in sufficient detail?
- Have the primary studies been combined or summarized appropriately?
- How sensitive are the results to changes in the way that the review is undertaken?
- Are judgements about preferences explicit?
- Are subgroup analyses interpreted cautiously?
- If there is 'no evidence of effect', is care taken not to interpret this as 'evidence of no effect'?

## The role of systematic reviews in evidence-based mental health nursing

- They are an important source of information for the development of clinical guidelines and best practice sheets.
- They are an efficient scientific technique.
- They can save professionals considerable time in accessing information.
- They can save money.

## Further reading

Greenhalgh T and Donald A. *Evidence Based Health Care Workbook for Individual and Group Learning.* BMJ Publishing Group: London, 2000.

Liberati A et al. The PRISMA statement for reporting systematic reviews and meta-analyses of studies that evaluate healthcare interventions: explanation and elaboration. *British Medical Journal* 2009; **339**: b2700.

NHS Centre for Reviews and Dissemination. *Undertaking Systematic Reviews of Research on Effectiveness: CRD's guidance for carrying out or commissioning reviews.* CRD Report 4, 2nd edn. NHS Centre for Reviews and Dissemination, University of York: York, 2001.

Sackett DL et al. (2000) *Evidence-Based Medicine: how to practice and teach EBM.* Churchill Livingstone: New York, 2000.

# Research

**Patrick Callaghan**

# The Triangle of Care (TOC)

### Introduction
The Triangle of Care is a guide for good practice in recognizing and working with carers as partners in care, published by the Carers Trust in 2010 and revised in 2013.[1] The 'triangle' refers to a therapeutic alliance between the service user, the professional, and the carer (see Figure 14.1 and Table 14.1).

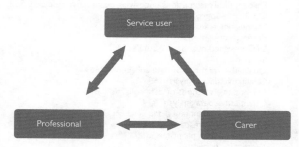

Fig. 14.1 The Triangle of Care.

Table 14.1 The six standards of the Triangle of Care[1]

| Standard number | Standard | Examples of good practice |
|---|---|---|
| 1 | Carers are essential to care and should be identified at first contact or as soon as possible thereafter | Carers' views and knowledge are sought, shared, used, and regularly updated to support treatment and recovery |
| 2 | Staff should be 'carer aware' and trained in carer engagement strategies | Staff should be aware of carers' needs and welcome carers' contribution<br>Staff require knowledge, training, and support |
| 3 | Policies and protocols with regard to confidentiality and sharing information with carers should be in place | Guidelines on confidentiality<br>Information release forms<br>Advance statement and protocols |
| 4 | There should be defined posts in each service with responsibility for carers | Carers' lead or champion<br>Carers' link delegated for each shift |
| 5 | Carers should have a formal introduction to the service and staff, and play an important role in care pathways | An introductory welcome letter from the team<br>Meeting with a named member of staff to discuss their views and opportunities for involvement<br>Induction and orientation to the ward<br>Carer information packs<br>Discharge planning and aftercare with support |
| 6 | Carer support services should be available | Carer support<br>Carer needs assessment<br>Family interventions |

**Reference**
1 Carers Trust. *The Triangle of Care. Carers included: a guide to best practice in mental health care in England.* Carers Trust: London, 2013.

# The research process

Research is the process of generating new knowledge through systematic enquiry governed by scientific principles.

## The purposes of research

- To improve practice.
- To defend practice.
- To increase the existing body of knowledge.
- To widen the repertoire of interventions.
- To improve cost-effectiveness.
- To provide evidence to support demands for extra resources.
- To satisfy academic or intellectual curiosity.
- To facilitate inter-professional collaboration.
- To earn or defend a professional status.

## The research process

This consists of:

- setting research questions(s), objective(s), and—where appropriate—hypotheses
- searching and retrieving literature
- reviewing the literature
- preparing a research proposal
- obtaining ethical approval
- accessing the research site
- collecting data
- handling and/or processing the collected data
- disseminating, diffusing, and implementing the research results.

## The five phases of research

*Conceptual phase*

This phase involves formulating the research problem, reviewing the related literature, defining a theoretical framework, and formulating hypotheses, research questions, or objectives.

*Design and planning*

This phase involves selecting the research design, identifying the sampling frame and the research sample, specifying methods, finalizing the research plan, obtaining ethical approval, conducting the pilot study, and making revisions to the original proposal if necessary.

*Empirical phase*

This phase involves collecting data and then preparing the data for analysis.

*Analytical phase*

This phase involves analysing the data and interpreting the results.

*Dissemination phase*

This phase involves communicating and implementing the findings of the research through evidence-based activities such as educational outreach visits and interactive educational meetings.

## Uses of research in mental health nursing

- Practice.
- Education.
- Service development.
- Management.
- Policy.

## Further reading

Gerrish K and Lacey A (eds). *The Research Process in Nursing*, 6th edn. Wiley-Blackwell: London, 2010.

Polit DF and Beck C. *Essentials of Nursing Research: appraising evidence for nursing practice*, 8th edn. Lippincott Williams & Wilkins: Philadelphia, PA, 2013.

Robson C. *Real World Research*, 3rd edn. John Wiley & Sons: Chichester, 2011.

# Philosophical assumptions underlying quantitative research

Quantitative approaches are used when researchers wish to test theory, other assumptions, and relationships between two or more variables. The quantitative research process usually follows predetermined stages.

## Empiricism

Often called 'British empiricism' (after the work of the British philosophers George Berkeley, David Hume, and John Locke), empiricism holds that knowledge derived from experience is more scientific and provides better evidence than knowledge derived from the senses or by the use of reason.

*Assumptions of empiricism*

- We should be sceptical about conclusions reached by the use of reason or the senses.
- Scrupulous (empirical) observation of human life allows us to develop laws about human behaviour.

*Critique of empiricism*

- It has led to more use of scientific methods to generate data.
- It has promoted the development of experimental methods in the health, human, and behavioural sciences.
- It undermines the role of reasoning, which may be useful for generating ideas to be tested empirically.
- Reason is necessary in order to understand the meaning and application of knowledge that is generated empirically.

## Logical positivism

Also called 'logical empiricism', logical positivism originates from the work of a group of philosophers—known as the Vienna Circle—in the 1920s. Whereas empiricism holds that knowledge is derived from personal experience, positivism holds that knowledge ultimately rests upon public experimental verification.

*Assumptions of positivism*

- Metaphysical rules are meaningless.
- All genuine knowledge can be expressed in a single language that is common to all sciences.
- Theories that cannot be tested are not scientific.
- The aim of science is to seek causality, not meaning.
- A theory is only scientific if it generates universal knowledge.
- There is an objective reality that can be studied, measured, and understood.

*Critique of positivism*

- It is reductionist (or focused?).
- It holds a narrow view of science.
- Few theories can generate universal knowledge.
- The application of positivism has led to significant (health) discoveries.

- Human behaviour involves meaningful intentions, expectations, and action.
- Different sciences have different languages—the language of social sciences differs from that of natural sciences.
- Reality can only be approximated, not fully understood.
- It has generated universal theories (e.g. relativity).

## Falsificationism

Falsificationism is derived from the work of Karl Popper, which was first published in 1935 (in German; it was first published in English in 1959), and is often referred to as postpositivism.[2]

*Assumptions of falsification*
- Theories derive from deductive testing of ideas.
- Refutability is at the heart of scientific reasoning.
- Falsification (proving something to be false), not verification, is crucial in science.

*Critique of falsificationism*
- Theories can never be truly established.
- Theory acceptance is tentative, whereas theory rejection can be decisive.
- Some well-established theories may have been rejected at birth.

## The relationship of empiricism, positivism, and falsificationism to health and social care research

Arguably, logical positivism no longer exists in its purest forms. Contemporary empiricism is more suited to health and social care research. It is characterized by identifying factors that are thought to be the key to understanding and explaining health and social phenomena, theory testing, and theory generation.

Contemporary empiricism, positivism, and falsificationism may be reflected in mental health nursing research by:
- research methods—including experimental designs, observations, and correlational designs
- developing empirical indicators of human behaviour
- theory development and testing
- building and strengthening the professional status of nursing.

The core differences between quantitative and qualitative approaches to research are summarized in Table 14.2. For a more detailed discussion of how each of these philosophies can be applied to mental health nursing research, the reader is referred to the paper by Gelo.[3]

## Conclusion

Researchers often treat quantitative and qualitative approaches as competing opposites in the battle for the supremacy of ideas and knowledge. The reality is that there are many sources of knowledge, and each has the potential to inform those with an open and critical mind.

**Table 14.2** Summary of the core differences between qualitative and quantitative approaches to research

| Criteria | Quantitative approach | Qualitative approach |
| --- | --- | --- |
| Use of positivism | Modified—contemporary empiricism | No |
| Acceptance of postmodern (PM) ideas | Unlikely—PM ideas may be seen as an attack on reason and truth | Increasing use |
| Capturing the individual's point of view | Yes, through reliable, objective measures | Yes, through detailed observation and interviewing |
| Examining the constraints of everyday life | Yes, through 'etic' perspectives based on probabilities derived from large data sets selected at random | Yes, through direct confrontation—the 'emic' perspective |
| Securing 'rich' descriptions | Less important | Valuable |

### References

2  Popper K. *The Logic of Scientific Discovery*. Routledge: London, 1959.
3  Gelo OCG. On research methods and their philosophical assumptions: 'raising the consciousness of researchers' again. *Psychotherapie & Sozialwissenschaft* 2012; **14**: 109–28.

### Further reading

Gortner SR. Nursing's syntax revisited: a critique of philosophies said to influence nursing theories. *International Journal of Nursing Studies* 1993; **30**: 477–88.

# Qualitative approaches to research

When researchers use qualitative approaches, they are usually collecting or analysing narrative data (words) in order to understand a social setting or phenomenon, without preconceived notions of what they may find.

## Qualitative research designs

- *Ethnography*—investigating meanings, patterns, and experiences in defined cultural groups.
- *Phenomenology*—exploring the lived experience or real-world experience of individuals.
- *Ethology*—investigating people's behaviour in a natural setting.
- *Grounded theory*—investigating social processes within a defined social setting.
- *Symbolic interaction*—studying the way in which people interact in social groups, and the sense people make of these settings.
- *Discourse analysis*—investigating the nature of written and verbal dialogue.

## Assessing quality in qualitative research approaches

'Credibility' is a term used in qualitative research to demonstrate the reliability, validity, and quality of research methods. It differs in many respects to the notion of reliability and the validity methods used in quantitative research.

## Factors that improve credibility in qualitative research

- Respondent validation or member checking.
- Triangulation of methods, data, investigators, and theories.
- Clear exposition of data collection methods.
- Clear exposition of the process of data analysis.
- Reflexivity—examining the role of the researcher in the outcomes.
- Attention to negative cases; avoiding holistic bias.

## Further reading

Denzin NK and Lincoln YS (eds). *The SAGE Handbook of Qualitative Research*, 4th edn. Sage Publications: Thousand Oaks, CA, 2011.

# Formulating research questions

The research process often begins with the development of research questions (see Table 14.3). This usually happens during the conceptual stage of the research process.

➔ The research process, p. 350.

## Sources of research questions

### Experience

Researchers will often have experience of the topic in which they are interested, and they may draw upon this experience to find research questions.

### Social issues

These are a useful source of research questions. Researchers will often consider a range of social issues, especially those that indicate significant social problems or concerns. For example, increased levels of antisocial behaviour by young people may be considered a significant social issue, and research might help to elucidate the nature and causes of such behaviour.

### Public health issues

These are issues that are often of concern to public health. For example, the increases in MRSA infection among people admitted to hospital or the rise of tuberculosis.

### Policy issues

These are issues that arise from government policies. For example, the National Service Framework for Mental Health provides a rich source of potential research questions.

### Theory

Nursing, health, and social care theories, or theories of human behaviour, are rich sources of research questions. For example, Peplau[4] argues that mental health nursing is an interpersonal process in which the nurse plays various roles—resource person, surrogate parent, and leader. Research questions arising from this theory could investigate whether Peplau's views can be substantiated by research or applied across all areas of mental health nursing.

Table 14.3 Examples of research problems and research questions

| Research problem | Research question |
| --- | --- |
| Unsure how young people experience mental health problems | How do young people experience mental health problems? |
| Limited evidence about the effects of ward rules and regulations on patients in acute psychiatric wards | What are the effects of ward rules and regulations on patients in acute psychiatric wards? |
| Lack of understanding about whether cognitive behavioural therapy (CBT) is more effective than interpersonal psychotherapy (IPT) in helping people to cope with depression | How does CBT compare with IPT in helping people to cope with depression? |

*External sources*
These include ideas suggested by others, who may be colleagues, experts in the field of interest, or service users.

## Developing and refining a research problem
- Select the problem.
- Narrow down the problem.
- Evaluate the problem.
- Evaluate the research problem.
- What is the significance of the problem?
- How researchable is the problem?
- How feasible is it to address the problem?

## Assessing the feasibility of research problems
Consider the following factors:
- time and timing
- availability of study participants
- cooperation of others
- facilities and equipment
- money
- experience of the researcher(s)
- ethical considerations.

## Reference
4 Peplau H. *Interpersonal Relations in Nursing: a conceptual frame of reference for psychodynamic nursing.* Springer Publishing Company: New York, 1991.

## Further reading
Polit DF and Beck C. *Essentials of Nursing Research: appraising evidence for nursing practice*, 8th edn. Lippincott Williams & Wilkins: Philadelphia, PA, 2013.
Robson C. *Real World Research*, 3rd edn. John Wiley & Sons: Chichester, 2011.

# Research designs

A research design is a description of the specific research approach employed by researchers. There are a variety of research designs, and the choice of design largely depends on the research questions. Some examples of commonly used research designs are described in this section.

## Quantitative research designs

*Randomized controlled trial (RCT) (also known as experimental design)*
Often called the 'gold standard' of quantitative designs, the RCT is used to test cause-and-effect relationships between at least two variables.

*Survey*
This involves collecting data in the form of questionnaires sent by post, structured face-to-face interviews, or telephone interviews.

*Single case study*
This is a highly structured study of one person.

*Comparative study*
This involves the comparison of at least two nominal groups.

*Factorial study*
This design involves the study of the relationship between multiple variables.

## Qualitative research designs

*Ethnography*
This is the study of people in their natural setting, through observation and interviews.

*Phenomenology*
This is the study of the lived experience or real-world experience of individuals, by means of unstructured or semi-structured interviews.

*Action research*
This involves the study of health and social care systems with a view to addressing identified problems. A researcher who is undertaking action research will work in collaboration with people inside the systems they are studying, using a variety of research methods.

There are other research designs—for example, historical research, symbolic interaction, or longitudinal designs. Some are only used within one research tradition, whereas others straddle both research traditions.
*Triangulated designs* involve the use of two or more methods in the same study.

## Further reading

Bowling A. *Research Methods in Health*, 3rd edn. Open University Press: Buckingham, 2009.
Denzin NK and Lincoln YS (eds). *The SAGE Handbook of Qualitative Research*, 4th edn. Sage Publications: Thousand Oaks, CA, 2011.

# Well-designed quantitative studies

The ultimate quality of quantitative research depends on the extent to which it minimizes threats to validity. 'Good' quantitative research designs are those that are appropriate to the research question and to the aims and objectives of the research, that lack bias, that are precise, and that have an appropriate statistical power.

## Categories of quantitative research designs

- Cross-sectional.
- Longitudinal.
- Comparative.
- Retrospective.
- Prospective.

## Types of quantitative research designs

- Experimental.
- Quasi-experimental.
- Solomon four group—essentially where there are two experimental groups and two control groups.
- Factorial.
- Repeated measures.
- RCTs.
- Time series.
- Single case.
- Correlational.
- Case study.
- Evaluation.
- Survey.
- Delphi method.
- Secondary analysis.
- Meta-analysis.
- Methodological.

## Threats to internal and external validity

### Internal validity

Internal validity occurs when the outcomes result only from the effect of the independent variable. Threats to internal validity arise from:

- lack of control of 'noise'
- the history of the subjects
- sample selection
- maturation of subjects
- effects of previous testing
- bias in research instruments
- response bias
- lack of adequate statistical power
- attrition or mortality—this is when participants withdraw from the study
- setting the significance level too high.

*Approaches to dealing with threats to internal validity*
- Better design.
- Homogeneity.
- Use of reliable and valid measures.
- Increasing the size of the population sampled.

*External validity*

External validity is the potential of the research to be generalized to other situations. Threats to external validity arise from:
- the Hawthorne effect, where participants respond simply because of the attention they receive from the researcher
- unrepresentative samples (number and quality)
- the novelty of new experiences for researchers and study participants alike
- the characteristics of the researcher
- measurement effects—that is, changes caused by simple exposure to the data collection methods.

*Approaches to dealing with threats to external validity*
- Standard protocols.
- Double-blind procedures.
- Supervision.
- Having an adequate sample that will allow detection of changes to be predicted with confidence.
- Having a representative sample.

## Controlling for 'noise'

In quantitative research designs it is important to control the variables that might have a causal or related effect on the research outcomes. This is known as 'noise'. Ways of controlling for 'noise' include:
- randomization
- repeated measures
- homogeneity
- blocking
- matching
- analysis of covariance (ANCOVA).

*Note:* measures to improve the internal validity of a study often unavoidably interfere with external validity. It may be necessary to accept this situation, as internal validity is more important.

## Further reading

Polit DF and Beck C. *Essentials of Nursing Research: appraising evidence for nursing practice*, 8th edn. Lippincott, Williams & Wilkins: Philadelphia, PA, 2013.
Robson C. *Real World Research*, 3rd edn. John Wiley & Sons: Chichester, 2011.

# Sampling

## What is sampling?

Sampling is the process of deciding on the number and characteristics of the people who will be invited to participate in a study. Sampling is a process of selecting part of a population to represent the entire population. Because the researcher may want to make comments about the entire population on the basis of the results obtained for their sample, that sample must be representative of the entire population.

There are two broad approaches to sampling:
- *Probability sampling*—where the researcher uses *random sampling* to select respondents.
- *Non-probability sampling*—where the researcher uses *non-random sampling*.

## Probability sampling

### Simple random sampling

Every member of the entire population has an equal chance of being selected. First, the entire eligible population—*the sampling frame*—is identified. Then the researcher randomly selects from this population—for example, by using random numbers, or pulling names out of a hat or card index. Simple random sampling may mean that the sample is not representative.

### Stratified random sampling

The researcher first divides the population into different groups, or strata. Then a sample is randomly selected from each group, making the sample more representative of the entire population.

### Cluster random sampling

This involves reducing large groups into small clusters (groups of similar things), and randomly selecting from within these clusters. This type of sampling is used to reduce the demands of surveying large groups, which might be time consuming, expensive, and unnecessary.

### Systematic random sampling

This involves selecting every nth person from a list or group. For example, if you need a sample size of 150 from a sampling frame of 40,000, you have to divide 40,000 by 150, which gives 266. Therefore every 266th person from your sampling frame would be selected until you reached 150.

## Non-probability sampling

### Convenience sampling

This uses the most conveniently available group of people. It is sometimes called 'opportunistic sampling', and may be used when it is not possible to use random sampling, or to save time. The use of convenience sampling is not likely to result in a representative sample.

*Quota sampling*
This involves sampling different groups, but not randomly. It is basically a combination of purposive and stratified sampling, but without random selection.

*Purposive sampling*
This is sometimes called judgemental sampling or theoretical sampling. The researcher uses their knowledge of the sample to select who should be included in the study. The sample is selected because it is felt that those particular individuals might be typical of the sampling frame.

*Snowball sampling*
In this sampling method, respondents refer someone they know to the researcher. The sample is selected on the basis of the researcher collecting contacts from respondents incrementally (the snowball effect).

## Important issues to consider when sampling
- Inclusion and exclusion criteria.
- Sample size.
- Attrition—where participants withdraw from the study.
- Bias—in responses and sampling methods.

## Steps involved in the sampling process
- Identify the target population.
- Identify the accessible population.
- Specify the eligibility criteria.
- Specify the sampling plan.
- Recruit the sample.

## Further reading
Gerrish K and Lacey A (eds) *The Research Process in Nursing*, 6th edn. Wiley-Blackwell: London, 2010.
Polit DF and Beck C. *Essentials of Nursing Research: appraising evidence for nursing practice*, 8th edn. Lippincott Williams & Wilkins: Philadelphia, PA, 2013.

# Qualitative methods of data collection

Observations and interviews are the data collection methods most commonly used in mental health nursing research. These methods are preferred because they allow greater insight into a person's experience and the meaning they attach to that experience.

## Observational methods

This method involves the systematic selection, observation, and recording of behaviour, events, and settings relevant to a research problem. Observations may be structured or unstructured. Structured observations are more likely to be used in quantitative studies.

## Characteristics that are observed

- Characteristics and conditions of individuals.
- Verbal and non-verbal behaviours.
- Activities.
- Skill attainment and performance.
- Environmental characteristics.

## Strengths of observational methods

- They are comprehensive.
- They create a more natural setting.
- They may validate other methods.
- They provide 'richer' data.

## Weaknesses of observational methods

- Observer bias and influence may occur.
- They create an artificial setting.
- They are intrusive.
- They are labour intensive.
- Training is required.
- They are costly.

## Strengths of interviews

- They provide high response rates.
- They may be more acceptable to participants.
- They provide opportunities to improve clarity.
- They allow a more in-depth discussion.
- Participants are less likely to miss questions.
- The order of the questions can be controlled.
- There is greater control over the participants—you know who has provided data.
- Supplementary data can be produced more readily.

## Weaknesses of interviews

- They are costly and time consuming.
- There is a lack of anonymity.
- Interviewer bias may occur.
- Participants have less control.
- They involve the use of expensive equipment such as digital recorders.
- They are more intrusive in that the researcher has an opportunity to probe more deeply into issues, which may be less possible with other methods such as questionnaires.
- They are not always as acceptable to participants.
- There is a possibility of response bias.

## Further reading

Denzin NK and Lincoln YS (eds). *The SAGE Handbook of Qualitative Research*, 4th edn. Sage Publications: Thousand Oaks, CA, 2011.

# Qualitative data analysis

The analysis of qualitative data requires clear thinking and attention to detail on the part of the analyst. In qualitative data analysis the researcher is like a research tool—there is a great need for reflection, sensitivity, awareness, and/or setting aside biases. There are many approaches to analysis, but most approaches have a number of features in common.

## The focus of qualitative analysis

The focus of qualitative analysis is on:
- the characteristics of language
- the discovery of regularities
- the comprehension of the meaning of text
- reflection.

## Types of qualitative data analysis

### Quasi-statistical methods

These involve the use of statistical procedures, such as counting how often forms of narrative data occur. Content analysis is an example of a quasi-statistical method.

### Template approaches

Themes and codes may be predetermined prior to the analysis and a template developed. The researcher then searches the data for evidence of these themes and codes. Matrix analysis is an example of a template approach.

### Editing approaches

These do not involve any predetermined themes and codes, only those based on the researcher's interpretation of the text. Grounded theory is an example of an editing approach.

### Immersion approaches

This approach is close to artistic interpretation, with little structure.

## Common features of qualitative data analysis

- Coding data.
- Adding comments.
- Identifying themes, categories, sequences, relationships, and differences between groups.
- Checking these themes with participants.
- Generating a small set of generalized themes that describe the consistencies from the analysis.
- Linking these generalized themes to theories.

## Further reading

Gerrish K and Lacey A (eds). *The Research Process in Nursing*, 6th edn. Wiley-Blackwell: London, 2010.
Miles MB and Huberman AM. *Qualitative Data Analysis*, 3rd edn. Sage Publications: Thousand Oaks, CA, 2013.
Robson C. *Real World Research*, 3rd edn. John Wiley & Sons: Chichester, 2011.

# Quantitative methods of data collection

Questionnaires, observations, and interviews are the most common data collection methods in mental health nursing research. Questionnaires are popular because they are easy to use and can collect research data from large samples spread over a wide geographical area. Researchers may design a questionnaire, modify a questionnaire designed by others, or use a questionnaire designed by others without amendment. Observation and interviews are often used because they allow a greater insight into a person's experience, and the meaning they attach to that experience.

## Questionnaires (e.g. Likert scales)

*Strengths of questionnaires*

- They are relatively cheap.
- They are easy to use.
- They are less time consuming for both the researcher and the respondent.
- They allow respondents to reply at their own convenience.
- They give respondents control—they can check their responses for accuracy.
- They provide greater confidentiality and anonymity for respondents.
- They avoid interviewer bias.
- They allow easier and faster data analysis.
- They are reliable—all of the respondents are asked the same questions.
- The researcher does not have to rely on memory, digital recorders, or note taking.

*Limitations of questionnaires*

- The respondents may be dishonest.
- Questionnaires have social desirability bias.
- The respondents' responses may be restricted.
- They reveal little about the context in which the responses were chosen.
- One cannot be certain that the person who returned the questionnaire is the respondent.
- Respondents may gauge the researcher's intention and respond accordingly.
- There is a high risk of non-responses.

A serious weakness of questionnaires is the risk of a low response rate. The following may help to improve your response rate:

- Estimate the response rate and make necessary allowances.
- Warn potential respondents in advance.
- Explain how the respondents were selected.
- Obtain sponsorship.
- Personalize the envelopes.
- Publicize the study.

- Offer incentives.
- Assure the respondents that confidentiality will be maintained.
- Issue reminders.
- Ensure anonymity.
- Enhance the appearance of the questionnaire.
- Shorten the length of the questionnaire if possible.
- Provide return envelopes.
- Highlight the interest of the topic to the respondent.
- Build a rapport with the respondents.

## Observational methods

These involve the systematic selection, observation, and recording of behaviour, events, and settings that are relevant to a research problem. Observations may be structured or unstructured, but the former are more likely in quantitative studies.

### What is observed?

- Characteristics and conditions of individuals.
- Verbal and non-verbal behaviours.
- Activities.
- Skill attainment and performance.
- Environmental characteristics.

### Strengths of observational methods

- They are comprehensive.
- They can create a more natural setting.
- They may validate other methods.
- They provide 'richer' data.

### Weaknesses of observational methods

- Observer bias and influence may occur.
- They can create an artificial setting.
- They are intrusive.
- They are labour intensive.
- Training is required.
- They are costly.

## Structured interviews

### Strengths of structured interviews

- High response rates.
- They may be more acceptable to participants.
- They allow opportunities to improve clarity.
- They allow a more in-depth discussion.
- Participants are less likely to miss questions.
- The order of the questions can be controlled.
- There is greater control over the participant—you know who has provided data.
- They can produce supplementary data more readily.

*Weaknesses of structured interviews*
- They are costly and time consuming.
- They lack anonymity.
- Interviewer bias may occur.
- Participants have less control.
- They involve the use of expensive equipment.
- They are more intrusive.
- They are not always as acceptable to participants.
- It is possible that participants may give dishonest answers or answer in a way designed to please the researcher.

## Further reading

Boynton PM and Greenhalgh T. Selecting, designing, and developing your questionnaire. *British Medical Journal* 2004; **328**: 1312–15.
Gerrish K and Lacey A (eds). *The Research Process in Nursing*, 6th edn. Wiley-Blackwell: London, 2010.
Parahoo K. Questionnaires: use, value and limitations. *Nurse Researcher* 1994; **1**: 4–11.

# Quantitative data analysis

This type of data analysis uses statistical procedures to give meaning to information collected during the research.

## Descriptive statistics

These are used to describe and merge data. The main descriptive statistics used are:

- measures of central tendency—mean, median, and mode
- distribution—standard deviation and range.

Numerical data may also be described using graphs, tables, or figures. It is important to know about level of measurement before you describe your data.

## Level of measurement

This is a system for categorizing different types of measures. There are four levels of measurement—nominal, ordinal, interval, and ratio. Although different measures may use different levels of measurement, it is possible to convert data to represent a different level of measurement. For example, if you request people's ages by using categories 21–30, and so on, this is nominal data, whereas if you ask people to state their age, this is interval data.

## Inferential statistics

These allow researchers to draw conclusions from their data. Broadly speaking there are three types of quantitative research design—surveys, correlational design, and experimental design. Within each of these designs the quantitative researcher usually tests relationships between variables.

## Statistical tests

A statistical test is an analytical procedure that allows a researcher to determine the likelihood that results obtained from a sample reflect true population results, according to the laws of probability.

*Reasons for using a statistical test*
- To determine whether you can generalize the results beyond the sample studied.
- To determine whether or not the results obtained are statistically significant.
- To determine whether you can reject the null hypothesis that states that the variables are not related.

*Factors that influence the choice of statistical test*
- Level of measurement.
- Sample size and sampling method.
- The degree of variance in responses to the dependent variable.
- The research design.
- The number of independent variables.
- The number of levels of the independent variables.

## Level of significance (probability level)

This is the level at which the researcher is prepared to reject or accept the null hypothesis. The level of significance is the probability of the researcher's results occurring by chance. It also gives information on the potential of research results to be generalized beyond the sample studied. The significance level is usually expressed as follows:

- $P < 0.05$—the researcher will reject the null hypothesis if the results are significant 95 times out of 100.
- $P < 0.01$—the researcher will reject the null hypothesis if the results are significant 99 times out of 100.
- $P < 0.10$—the researcher will reject the null hypothesis if the results are significant 90 times out of 100.

For example, suppose that a researcher compares CBT with supportive psychotherapy (SP) for treating the negative symptoms of schizophrenia. Imagine that the researcher analysed the results of this study and found that CBT was more effective than SP in reducing negative symptoms, and the results were statistically significant at $P < 0.05$. This means that there is a 5 in 100 chance that the negative symptoms were reduced by something other than CBT.

## Further reading

Gerrish K and Lacey A (eds). *The Research Process in Nursing*, 6th edn. Wiley-Blackwell: London, 2010.
Heavey E. *Statistics for Nursing: a practical approach*, 2nd edn. Jones & Bartlett Learning: Burlington, MA, 2014.
Kanji GK. *100 Statistical Tests*, 3rd edn. Sage Publications: London, 2006.
Polit DF and Beck C. *Essentials of Nursing Research: appraising evidence for nursing practice*, 8th edn. Lippincott Williams & Wilkins: Philadelphia, PA, 2013.

# Key issues in quantitative data analysis

### Selection of an appropriate statistical test

Before running a statistical test on research data, you must check that your research design meets the requirements of the test you propose to use. There are two broad types of statistical tests—parametric and non-parametric. Within each of these types there are many different tests. Parametric tests are the strongest tests, and most researchers prefer to use these tests on their data where possible. However, the rules for running parametric tests are stricter than those for non-parametric tests.

### Parametric versus non-parametric tests

The research community has debated at length how strict one should be in applying the rule regarding level of measurement for the use of parametric tests. You can apply both parametric and non-parametric tests to ordinal data. If the results are contradictory then you should report the results of the non-parametric test.

*Requirements for using parametric tests*

Your data should meet the following requirements before you may use a parametric test:

- Your level of measurement should be *interval* at least (with the above in mind).
- Your scores should be normally distributed.
- The variability in your data should be homogeneous.

When designing the study, you need to pay particular attention to the level of measurement of the instruments that you use, and of the demographic data that you collect. Normal distribution and variance can be tackled by sampling techniques that maximize the representativeness of your sample.

### Statistical power analysis

This is a procedure for reducing the likelihood of making a type 2 error (see p. 377). It determines the probability of obtaining a significant result. There are four components of a power analysis. The researcher must know at least three of these beforehand. These components are:

- level of significance (see p. 377)
- population effect size
- sample size
- power.

Researchers use power analysis to determine the sample size needed to demonstrate significant results and to determine the power of a statistical test. Achieving statistical power is not simply a matter of increasing sample size. It can also be achieved by ensuring that treatment conditions of an independent variable are different from control conditions, selecting dependent variables that are realistically related to independent variables, and the timing of measuring a dependent variable.

## Level of significance

This is the level at which you are prepared to reject or accept the null hypotheses. The level of significance is really the probability of your results occurring by chance, or as a result of your research design. It will also provide information on the potential of your findings to be generalized beyond your sample. Obviously, the lower the level of significance the more likely you are to reject the null hypotheses. In most quantitative social and behavioural science research, the level of significance is normally set at 5% or $P < 0.05$.

## Type 1 and type 2 errors

A type 1 error is when you say that two variables were related to one another when in fact they were not. This is most likely to occur when the researcher fails to detect differences between the groups at the beginning of the research. A type 2 error is made when the researcher concludes that the variables are not related, when in fact they are. When these errors occur, differences that appear between the groups at the end of the research are interpreted as arising from the research design, whereas in fact they were apparent from the outset of the research. Type 1 and type 2 errors will mislead people and can have serious consequences (e.g. in an RCT testing the effect of a new drug).

*Factors that help to avoid type 1 and type 2 errors*
- Adequate sample size.
- A representative sample.
- An appropriate research design.
- A homogeneous sample.

## Establishing the psychometric status of research measures

This may be the first stage of analysis after your descriptive statistics. It will involve calculating coefficients to determine the reliability and concurrent validity of your measure(s).

*Types of analyses*
There are two broad categories of quantitative data analyses:
- *Bivariate analyses* are tests that:
  - look for differences between groups as defined by one variable, on scores on another variable
  - test associations (relationships or correlations) between scores on two variables.
- *Multivariate analyses* are tests that:
  - look for differences between two or more groups on a number of dependent variables
  - test associations between scores on a number of variables.

## Further reading

Heavey E. *Statistics for Nursing: a practical approach*, 2nd edn. Jones & Bartlett Learning: Burlington, MA, 2014.

Kanji GK. *100 Statistical Tests*, 3rd edn. Sage Publications: London, 2006.

Polit DF and Beck C. *Essentials of Nursing Research: appraising evidence for nursing practice*, 8th edn. Lippincott Williams & Wilkins: Philadelphia, PA, 2013.

# Ethical issues in research

All human behaviour occurs in the context of ethical and moral codes, and the practice of research is no different in this respect. Researchers must ensure that they are adhering to universally acknowledged ethical principles—such as those described in the Helsinki Declaration of 1952—in the conduct of their research. It is these principles that are described here.

## The principle of beneficence

Research should yield benefits. Mental health nursing research should ultimately benefit people who use mental health services. People who participate in research must be protected from harm and exploitation. An assessment of the risk:benefit ratio should help researchers and those who govern the conduct of research to ensure that the principle of beneficence is upheld.

## The principle of respect for human dignity

Researchers must respect the rights of participants and ensure that their dignity is upheld at all times during the research process. Participants have the right to self-determination, and should be fully informed of what researchers require of them, and why.

## The principle of justice

People who participate in research have the right to fair treatment and privacy.

## Informed consent

Researchers must not enrol people in research who have not given their informed consent to participate. To be fully informed, potential participants must know their status, the purpose of the study, the type of data that will be collected, the nature of the commitment expected of them, how they were selected for participation, what exactly they must do, and the potential benefits and risks of participating. Participants should know that their consent is voluntary and that they can withdraw from the research at any time with impunity, and that alternatives to treatment that might have been given for research purposes will be available to them if they withdraw from the research. Participants should also be given information on who to contact to discuss the research and their participation. They should be informed that all information they provide to researchers is confidential, unless this information threatens the health and safety of others.

## Working with vulnerable people

There are additional safeguards when research includes participants who are classed as vulnerable. Vulnerable groups include children, people with learning or physical disabilities, mental illness, or terminal illness, pregnant women, and those who are institutionalized.

## External review and approval

Researchers must comply with the ethical procedures of their respective governments. Research involving humans or animals should not be conducted until a Research Ethics Committee has approved it. The Department of Health in England requires that researchers adhere to its research governance framework (which can be found on its website at 🔗 www.dh.gov.uk).

## Further reading

Fouka G and Mantzorou M. What are the major ethical issues in conducting research? Is there a conflict between research ethics and the nature of nursing? *Health Science Journal* 2011; 5: 3–14.

Polit DF and Beck C. *Essentials of Nursing Research: appraising evidence for nursing practice*, 8th edn. Lippincott Williams & Wilkins: Philadelphia, PA, 2013.

Royal College of Nursing. *Research Ethics: RCN guidance for nurses*. Royal College of Nursing: London, 2009.

# Writing research proposals

### General points
- Write in the future tense.
- Tailor the proposal to the guidelines.
- The structure will be similar to that of a research report.
- Be succinct and focused.
- A proposal may change after consultation with your supervisor or advisers.

### Stages involved in writing a research proposal
- Abstract—a synopsis of the whole proposal.
- Significance of the proposed research.
- Background or literature review.
- Aims and objectives.
- Research questions or hypotheses (if appropriate).
- Methods.
- Design.
- Sample and sampling.
- Data collection.
- Procedure.
- Data analysis.
- Dissemination.
- Ethical issues.

### Establishing the significance of the proposed study
- Relate the study to deficits in the existing literature.
- Relate the study to policy issues and recommendations (local, national, or international).
- Highlight innovations (e.g. of topic or methods).
- Target the proposal to the interests of the funding body.
- Show clearly how the proposed research will improve practice, education, management, and research.
- Describe its contribution to theory.
- Describe its general applicability.

### Background
- Review the important existing literature—be selective.
- Show how the proposed research builds upon or extends existing work.
- Mount a coherent, convincing argument for the proposed research that is obvious to the reader.

### Aims and objectives
- Be specific.
- Be focused.
- Objectives must be achievable.
- Provide clear criteria against which the proposed methods can be assessed.

Research aims, objectives, questions, or hypotheses should be:
- clear
- succinct
- achievable
- specific
- focused
- related to methods.

## Design
- Describe the design.
- Justify the design.
- Adhere to criteria for well-designed studies (e.g. CONSORT statement).
- Describe the sample and sampling procedure.
- Describe the sample characteristics and size.
- Describe how the sample is to be accessed.
- Describe the determination of sample size.
- Describe the sampling method.
- Ensure that the sample is representative—use probability sampling if possible.
- Consider sampling issues for specific research approaches (e.g. focus groups, action research).
- Describe the data collection.
- Describe and justify the data collection methods.
- Address issues of reliability, validity, and credibility.
- Ensure that the methods can be independently verifiable.

## Procedure
- Describe in detail how attrition is dealt with (e.g. setting, protocols).
- Include the pilot study.

## Data analysis
- Describe in detail the proposed analysis.
- Describe exactly what the analysis will yield.
- Ensure systematic analysis.
- Address issues of reducing bias.
- Describe how to resolve differences in interpretation if more than one person is analysing the data.

## Dissemination
- Describe dissemination in detail.
- Differentiate diffusion from dissemination.
- State how to implement the findings.

## Identify ethical issues raised by the proposed research
- State how ethical probity will be ensured.
- Ethical approval is almost always required.
- Adhere to the Research Governance Framework.

## Further reading
Gerrish K and Lacey A (eds). *The Research Process in Nursing*, 6th edn. Wiley-Blackwell: London, 2010.
Polit DF and Beck C. *Essentials of Nursing Research: appraising evidence for nursing practice*, 8th edn. Lippincott Williams & Wilkins: Philadelphia, PA, 2013.

# Writing for publication

Many mental health nurses publish work in a variety of outlets, such as journals, books, and online. The publication may be a research report, a clinical case study, or an opinion piece. Getting published is a competitive and demanding process. The following information may increase your chances of getting your work published.

## Developing writing skills

- The art of writing is about simplicity and clarity.
- Read examples of excellent writing—and not just academic writing.
- Practise with short pieces.
- Use critical readers, and seek feedback.
- Use manuals (e.g. *The Writer's Manual*[5]).
- Use software packages.
- Start at a basic level and then progress to more complex pieces.

## Clarifying the focus of the paper

- Plan the paper.
- Have a succinct introduction.
- Remind yourself of the aim of the paper.
- Stick to the aim.
- Use section headings.
- Make the conclusion succinct.

## Writing a research paper

*Introduction and literature review*

- Evaluate previous work.
- Identify knowledge gaps in previous work.
- Describe how your work addresses gaps in previous work.

*Methods*

- Structure this into sections, following the format or design of the particular publication.
- Sample—describe the sample and sampling methods.
- Measures and data collection methods—state what your data collection methods were.
- Procedure—describe exactly how the research was carried out.
- Data analysis—describe how the data were analysed.
- Results—report the results.

*Communicating research results*

Follow the sequence of aims, objectives, and hypotheses if appropriate:

- Use illustrations.
- Avoid jargon—state exactly what the results mean in lay terms.
- Give examples—use direct quotes.
- Summarize the results if they are lengthy.
- Use correct grammar.

## General tips on using English correctly
- Do not use double negatives.
- Make each pronoun agree with its antecedent.
- Do not dangle participles.
- Do not use unnecessary commas.
- Verbs must agree with their subject.
- Do not use sentence fragments.
- Try not to split infinitives.
- Use apostrophes correctly.
- Always read what you have written to see if you have left any words out.
- Correct spelling is essential.

## Reference
5  Cook R. *The Writer's Manual: a step-by-step guide for nurses and other health professionals*. Radcliffe Medical Press: Oxford, 1999.

## Further reading
Holland K and Watson R (eds). *Writing for Publication in Nursing and Healthcare: getting it right*. John Wiley & Sons: London, 2012.

Lester JD and Lester JD Jr. *Writing Research Papers: a complete guide*, 14th edn. Pearson: New York, 2013.

Turabian KL. *A Manual for Writers of Term Papers, Theses and Dissertations*, 7th edn. University of Chicago Press: Chicago, IL, 2007.

# Using research to improve practice

Mental health nursing is about promoting mental health, and caring for people using mental health services. The aim is to help people to recover their ability to live relatively free from ill health. Mental health nursing research is about providing an evidence base to support the activities of mental health nurses and others doing similar work. There is an overwhelming source of evidence-based information that nurses can use in their work. However, there are key skills required in using this evidence to improve practice, not least of which is the ability to evaluate published research.

The term 'evaluate' means to judge the worth or value of something. Evaluation requires a balanced critique during which you will identify the strengths and weaknesses of published evidence. The Critical Appraisal Skills Programme (CASP) website[6] has checklists for evaluating different types of research reports, and is an indispensable source of useful information for evaluating published research.

## General tips on evaluating published research

- Be as objective as possible.
- Do not insult the author(s) or question their competence.
- Be reasonable in your critique.
- Give specific examples of the strengths and limitations of the paper.
- Be sensitive when making negative statements—put yourself in the author's shoes.
- Try to justify your criticisms.
- Suggest alternatives.

## Getting research into practice

*What works?*
- Academic detailing—lectures.
- Opinion leaders—influential and credible individuals.
- Audit and feedback.
- Reminder systems.
- Patient-mediated interventions.

*Consistently effective interventions*
- Educational outreach visits.
- Reminders.
- Multifaceted interventions (e.g. two or more of audit and feedback, reminders, local consensus processes, and marketing).
- Interactive educational meetings.

*Interventions of variable effectiveness*
- Audit and feedback.
- Local opinion leaders.
- Local consensus processes.
- Patient-mediated interventions.

*Interventions that have little or no effect*
- Educational materials.
- Didactic educational meetings.

## The experience of putting evidence into practice

*Factors related to likelihood of success*
- Sufficient resources (i.e. time, money, and skills).
- Benefits to frontline staff from the proposed change.
- Enough of the right people are on board early enough.
- Interactive approach linking research clearly to practice.

*Key lessons*
- Expect to take several years.
- Successful implementation requires pragmatism and flexibility.
- Start small and build incrementally.
- Use what is already there.
- Target enthusiasts first.

*Outcomes*
- Better relationships.
- Improved knowledge, systems, and skills.
- Practice change.
- Improved patient care.

## Reference

6   Critical Appraisal Skills Programme (CASP) website. ℘ www.casp-uk.net

## Further reading

Bero LA et al. Closing the gap between research and practice: an overview of systematic reviews of interventions to promote the implementation of research findings. *British Medical Journal* 1998; **317**: 465–8.

Boaz A, Baeza J and Fraser A. Effective implementation of research into practice: an overview of systematic reviews of the health literature. *BMC Research Notes* 2011; **4**: 212. ℘ www.biomed-central.com/content/pdf/1756-0500-4-212.pdf

Gerrish K and Lacey A (eds). *The Research Process in Nursing*, 6th edn. Wiley-Blackwell: London, 2010.

Greenhalgh T. *How to Read a Paper: the basics of evidence-based medicine*. BMJ Books: London, 2010.

Wye L and McClenahan J. *Getting Better with Evidence: experiences of putting evidence into practice*. The King's Fund: London, 2000.

# Mixed methods research

### Introduction

Mixed methods research combines two or more data collection or data analysis methods in one study, and is an increasingly popular research method in nursing and health sciences research. The combination of quantitative and qualitative methods is the most common form of mixed methods research. However, using combinations of quantitative or qualitative methods also counts as mixed methods (see Tables 14.4 and 14.5).

Table 14.4 Different types of mixed methods designs[7]

| Design | Features | Example |
|--------|----------|---------|
| Explanatory sequential design | Phase 1: quantitative methods, followed by Phase 2: qualitative methods. The qualitative methods seek to explain the quantitative results | Quantitative observations of staff–resident interactions and qualitative interviews to explore reasons for the interaction levels observed[8] |
| Exploratory sequential design | Phase 1: qualitative methods are followed by Phase 2: quantitative methods. The quantitative methods seek to test the findings from phase 1 | Creating and validating a measure of organizational assimilation[9] |
| Embedded design | A qualitative strand is added to a quantitative study, or vice versa | Using an RCT to test a youth mentoring intervention with interviews to capture the participants' experiences of the intervention |
| Convergent parallel design | Quantitative and qualitative methods are used simultaneously, the data are merged, and the results are compared | Investigating concordance and discordance between physicians and patients about depression[10] |
| Transformative design | Using different methods guided by a transformative theoretical framework | Quantitatively identifying whether men and women have different social capital profiles, and using interviews to explain why women participate more in social and community activities within a feminist theoretical framework[11] |
| Multiphase design | A study that has multiple phases and uses quantitative and/or qualitative methods in different phases | Creating and validating culturally appropriate psychological measures, and developing and evaluating culturally appropriate interventions[12] |

Table 14.5 Strengths and limitations of mixed methods designs[13,14]

| Strengths | Limitations |
| --- | --- |
| Allow better validity as different methods can corroborate each other | The commensurability or incompatibility issue—can one be a positivist and an interpretivist at the same time? Mixed methods research often combines methods underpinned by different epistemologies that have different views of the nature of reality |
| Offer a deeper understanding of the issue under investigation | |
| Limitations of single approaches might be extinguished | Mixed methods undermine the possibility of developing expertise in a particular research method |
| Answer research questions that cannot be answered by other designs | The use of 'pragmatic' epistemologies that often underpin mixed methods projects fails to address deeper questions of practicality (e.g. practical for what and for whom?) |
| Explanations of findings are better | Requires knowledge of different methods that may mean larger research teams, thus increasing the cost of the research |

## References

7  Cresswell JW and Plano Clark VL. Designing and Conducting Mixed Methods Research, 2nd edn. London: Sage Publications, 2011.

8  Lau MH, Callaghan P, Twinn SF and Goodfellow B. The nursing gaze: power relations in a study of nurse–resident interactions in learning disability. Journal of Psychiatric and Mental Health Nursing 2007; 14: 346–55.

9  Myers KK and Ostzel JG. Exploring the dimensions of organisation assimilation: creating and validating a measure. Communication Quarterly 2003; 51: 438–57.

10  Wittink MN, Barg FK and Gallo JJ. Unwritten rules of talking to doctors about depression: integrating qualitative and quantitative methods. Annals of Family Medicine 2006; 4: 302–9.

11  Hodgkin S. Telling it all: a story of women's social capital using a mixed methods approach. Journal of Mixed Methods Research 2008; 2: 296–316.

12  Nastasi BK et al. Mixed methods in intervention research: theory to adaptation. Journal of Mixed Methods Research 2007; 1: 164–82.

13  Small ML. How to conduct a mixed methods study: recent trends in a rapidly growing literature. Annual Review of Sociology 2011; 37: 57–86.

14  Doyle L, Brady AM and Byrne G. An overview of mixed methods research. Journal of Research in Nursing 2009; 14: 175–85.

# Liaison mental health services

**Sarah Eales**

# Liaison mental health services

Liaison mental health services (LMHS) provide support to non-mental health practitioners and services. They aim to meet the psychological and mental health needs of patients who are receiving primary treatment for a non-mental health problem. They increasingly offer services in emergency departments to patients whose presenting problem is one of mental distress. It is estimated that up to 65% of medical inpatients have psychiatric symptoms.

## Evolution of liaison mental health services

Liaison mental health nursing was first developed in the USA. Liaison nurses were clinical specialists, offering support and education for general hospital nurses. They also provided care direct to patients and families.

Liaison mental health nursing in the UK developed in the 1990s. The government's concern to reduce suicide rates provided the impetus for the development of services in emergency departments and specific self-harm provision. Recent emphasis on 24-hour access to support for anyone with a mental health problem further increased the emergency department provision. Recent developments include the Rapid Assessment Interface and Discharge (RAID) service, which is a multidisciplinary model of 24-hour provision. The RAID model has become popular with commissioners because initial evaluations indicate that it can bring significant cost savings to the general hospital.[1]

## Structure of services

There are numerous models of LMHS. Liaison nurses usually work as part of a team that includes some or all of the following professionals:

- psychiatrists
- social workers
- psychologists
- occupational therapists.

There is no strong evidence to support one particular model of LMHS over another.

Service provision ranges from 9 a.m. to 5 p.m. Monday to Friday to 24-hour services that are provided 365 days of the year.

Liaison nurses work across all age ranges. However, adult services are more common than older adult or child and adolescent services. The RAID model advocates the joining together of adult and older adult services for maximum effectiveness.

➔ Assessment of children and adolescents, p. 146.

## Evaluation of services

The majority of published information about LMHS is descriptive. However, there is evidence that LMHS based in emergency departments ease the burden on general emergency department staff, help service users to access mental health services, and reduce the re-admission rates of people with mental health problems. There is also evidence that general hospital nurses value the responsiveness and the ease of access of liaison nursing services. The RAID model has shown positive outcomes in reducing length of stay, re-admission rates, and, most recently, admission via the emergency department.

## Reference

1 Tadros G et al. Impact of an integrated rapid response psychiatric liaison team on quality improvement and cost savings: the Birmingham RAID model. *Psychiatric Bulletin* 2013; **37**: 4–10.

## Further reading

Callaghan P, Eales S, Coats T and Bowers L. A review of the structure, process and outcome of liaison mental health services. *Journal of Psychiatric and Mental Health Nursing* 2003; **10**: 155–65.

Fossey M and Parsonage M. *Outcomes and Performance in Liaison Psychiatry*. Centre for Mental Health: London, 2014. &#x1F516; www.centreformentalhealth.org.uk/pdfs/Outcomes_and_perf_in_LP.pdf

Parsonage M and Fossey M (eds). *Economic Evaluation of a Liaison Psychiatry Service*. Centre for Mental Health: London, 2011. &#x1F516; http://socialwelfare.bl.uk/subject-areas/services-client-groups/adults-mental-health/centreformentalhealth/economic111.aspx

Parsonage M, Fossey M and Tutty C. *Liaison Psychiatry in the Modern NHS*. Centre for Mental Health: London, 2012. &#x1F516; www.centreformentalhealth.org.uk/pdfs/liaison_psychiatry_in_the_modern_NHS_2012.pdf

# The process of liaison mental health care

Liaison mental health nursing can take many forms. The most common is accepting a referral from another discipline, where there is a concern that the patient is showing signs of mental distress. This might be a known mental health problem, a psychological reaction to trauma, or a person with a suspected mental health problem presenting to the emergency department.

## A model for service provision

Liaison mental health nurses usually offer a range of services, not just the assessment and treatment of individual patients.

Caplan[2] identified the following models of liaison mental health service provision:

- *Client-centred service*—the direct assessment and treatment of a referred patient. Education is a secondary concern.
- *Programme-centred administrative service*—this includes involvement in planning service delivery advice on drawing up policies to assist nurses with one-to-one observation in a general hospital setting.
- *Consultee-centred service*—this involves working with the staff. Education is the primary concern here, rather than the individual patient. Nurses may lack the knowledge, skills, or confidence necessary to work with a patient who has a mental health problem.
- *Consultee-centred administrative service*—this involves ongoing support to maintain the mental health aspects of service delivery (e.g. follow-up visits to a ward or unit to review the implementation of training).

Client-centred and consultee-centred care are the most frequently provided services.

→ Person-centredness, p. 284.

## The process of liaison mental health care

When a patient is referred to the nurse, that nurse should establish the reason for referral, the presenting complaint, any evidence of risk behaviour, and the expected outcome from the perspective of the referrer. The patient's consent for the referral should always be obtained except in emergency situations.

Once the referral has been accepted, the nurse should undertake the following:

- *Gathering information*—obtain background information, including information from the GP and, where relevant, the patient's mental health team. Friends and relatives may have important information on the development of the problem, and the patient's mental health history.
- *Assessment*—undertake a thorough psychosocial assessment. It is important to consider the patient's perception of the problem and its cause. A mental state examination and a thorough risk assessment should be given a high priority in the assessment process (→ Mental health assessment, p. 36).

- *Formulation*—formulate a summary of the problems, including identification of current and potential risk, and triggers that lead to an increase in risk (➲ Risk, p. 163).
- *Treatment*—identify a treatment plan, taking time to discuss the options with the referrer and the patient before making a decision. Treatment may include referral to other mental health or substance misuse services. Short-term supportive counselling and brief cognitive behavioural therapy may be provided by the liaison nurse (➲ Cognitive behavioural therapy, p. 106; ➲ Motivational interviewing, p. 72).
- *Follow-up*—ongoing monitoring and treatment may be required. Repeating the mental state examination will help to determine the effectiveness of treatment and the reduction in symptoms.
- *Communication*—having identified whether a problem is present, the nature of any risk, and the treatment plan, it is important to ensure that the patient, the referrer, and any other relevant professionals are aware of the outcome of the assessment (➲ Interpersonal communication, p. 54).

**Reference**

2 Caplan G. *The Theory and Practice of Mental Health Consultation*. Tavistock Publications: London, 1970.

# Liaison mental health nursing competencies

Liaison mental health nurses may hold responsibility for decisions to admit or discharge patients. They are likely to be senior clinical nurses banded at Level 7. Working in the general hospital setting, they can be called to see patients whose primary problem is outside their specialist area. Good relationships within different specialisms are of paramount importance to ensure an understanding of the patient's primary problem.

There are a number of competencies of liaison mental health nursing, including effective documentation, that are common to mental health nurses in other areas, while others are specific to liaison mental health nursing.

## Competencies

Liaison nurses need to be competent to undertake work in the following areas:
- admission and discharge of patients
- assessment and management of risk and self-harm
- providing nursing advice on medication
- patients with complex or challenging presentations
- advice on legal and ethical issues, including capacity to consent (⮕ Assessing capacity to consent, p. 398)
- treatment appropriate to the general hospital setting, including managing dual medical–psychological presentations and psychiatric emergencies
- patients with specific physical disorders, including knowledge of the psychological morbidity associated with specific physical disorders
- patients with specific physical and psychosomatic disorders (⮕ Working with specific physical and psychosomatic disorders, p. 396)
- substance misuse, including identification of symptoms of withdrawal (⮕ People with substance misuse problems, p. 94)
- working across the lifespan, from perinatal care through childhood and adolescence, adulthood, and into older adulthood
- working with people with learning disabilities, particularly in supporting communication in treatment decision making and managing challenging presentations
- maintaining accurate records, documentation, and report writing, including preparation of discharge summaries (⮕ Writing and keeping records of care, p. 36)
- evaluation of liaison mental health nursing interventions.

## Further reading

Eales S, Wilson N and Waghorn J. A Competence Framework for Liaison Mental Health Nursing. London Liaison Mental Health Nurses' Special Interest Group: London, 2014. Unpublished document.
Harrison A. *The Role of the Nurse in Liaison Psychiatry*. Cambridge University Press: Cambridge, 2007.

# Working with specific physical and psychosomatic disorders

Nurses in a general hospital may require assistance in managing the psychological consequences of physical health problems. Nurses may be fearful of mental health problems—they may feel that they lack the knowledge and skills to meet psychological needs, or that they simply do not have the time to address them. Some patients present with physical symptoms for which no underlying physical cause can be identified; frequently these patients are suffering from a psychosomatic disorder. Liaison nurses have a role in the education of the nursing staff, assessment, planning, and treatment of comorbidity and psychosomatic illness.

## Epidemiology

Illnesses such as HIV and end-stage renal failure have a high incidence of accompanying psychological needs. Over 10% of medical admissions are for deliberate self-harm. Depression is evident in around 25–45% of general hospital patients. Approximately 1 in 10 patients who are admitted for an acute condition will have an acute confusional state accompanying their medical condition. Up to 50% of symptoms in an outpatient department may be unexplained by physical causes.

## Adjustment reactions and depression

It is quite usual to experience some psychological distress when in hospital. A change of environment, the absence of friends and relatives, and a concern about the treatment and prognosis can all lead to stress, anxiety, and fear.

The liaison nurse needs to educate and assist the general hospital team in how to distinguish between a normal reaction and an abnormal one. Prolonged problems in adjusting to physical illness may lead to depression, the most common mental illness. The liaison nurse has a key role in assessing, identifying, and recommending treatment for depression. They cannot rely on normal indicators such as sleep disturbance and loss of appetite, as these may be present as a consequence of the physical health problem. Untreated depression may delay recovery, interfere with activity such as physiotherapy, and prolong the physical illness. Symptoms such as withdrawal, pessimism, and guilt may be better indicators of depression in patients with physical health problems. The Hospital Anxiety and Depression Scale (HADS) is a validated tool for use in assessment.

## Acute confusional states (delirium)

Symptoms of acute confusion include:
- disorientation with regard to time and place
- psychotic symptoms, such as paranoia and hallucinations
- challenging behaviour.

Acute confusion will have an underlying physical cause—for example, infections (e.g. chest infection, urinary tract infection), constipation, or hypoxia.

The presentation may appear to indicate a psychiatric disorder, but the onset is usually very rapid rather than incremental. Liaison nurses need to be able to identify acute confusion and help the general nursing team to manage the symptoms while the underlying physical cause is treated.

### Further reading

Royal College of Psychiatrists. *Liaison psychiatry for every acute hospital: integrated mental and physical healthcare*. CR183. RCPsych: London, 2013. ℘ www.rcpsych.ac.uk/usefulresources/publications/collegereports/cr/cr183.aspx

# Assessing capacity to consent

→ Assessing mental capacity, p. 240

Every patient has the legal and ethical right to decide whether to enter into a particular type of care or treatment. The only exception is under specific sections of the Mental Health Act 2007 (see Chapter 8).

Consent may be written, verbal, or non-verbal, depending on the circumstances. The person who will be undertaking a procedure must obtain the patient's consent, and remains responsible for this. There are very few exceptions to this requirement to obtain consent. The Department of Health and each local health trust will have specific guidance on obtaining consent. The liaison nurse may be asked to assist in the assessment of capacity and/or in the gaining of consent.

## Principles of consent

The patient must:
- have the capacity to make the decision
- be provided with enough information to enable them to make the decision
- not be acting under duress.

All adults are in the first instance presumed to have capacity. An attempt should be made to obtain consent from every patient for all interventions. If the patient is unable to consent, treatment may still be given in the patient's 'best interests'.

No one can consent on behalf of an adult patient, although when a patient lacks capacity their friends and relatives may be able to assist the professional in making a 'best-interest' decision, and the patient's wishes when they previously had capacity (advance directives) should be reasonably honoured. The decision must be free from discrimination. Disagreement within the multidisciplinary team about 'best-interests' treatment and care will often lead to a request for a legal review of the issue.

## Assessment of capacity to consent

To assess capacity, the liaison nurse must be certain that the patient:
- can comprehend and retain the information needed to make a decision
- is able to use and weigh that information in the decision-making process.[3]

The National Institute for Health and Care Excellence (NICE) guidelines on self-harm[3] break this assessment down further. To demonstrate capacity to give or withhold consent, the individual should be able to:
- understand in simple language what the treatment is, its purpose and nature, and why it is being proposed
- understand its principal benefits, risks, and alternatives
- understand in broad terms what will be the consequences of not receiving the proposed treatment
- retain the information for long enough to make an effective decision
- believe the information
- weigh up the information
- make a free choice.

Patients frequently refuse to give consent because they do not understand the proposed treatment, and would benefit from further information. Refusal of treatment does not indicate a lack of capacity. Capacity may fluctuate in a patient, and for each procedure, lack of capacity should not be assumed.

Detailed documentation of any assessment and the decisions made is extremely important. The local health trust will have forms that need to be completed.

## Deprivation of liberty safeguards (DOLS)

DOLS are an important part of the Mental Capacity Act (MCA), and were developed to ensure that vulnerable people living in residential homes, supported living settings, and hospitals are not deprived of their liberty unless this is in their best interests. Vulnerable people are those aged 18 years or over who have a mental health problem, including dementia, and who *do not* have mental capacity to make their own decisions.

Under the MCA a person lacks capacity when they:
- do not understand information given to them
- cannot retain the information long enough to make a decision
- cannot weigh up information and understand the consequences of decisions
- cannot communicate their decision by whatever means available.

Depriving someone of their liberty requires a deprivation of liberty authorization, but this cannot be used with a person unless they lack capacity. DOLS do not apply to someone detained under the Mental Health Act.

### The safeguards
These include:
- providing the person with a representative or advocate
- giving the person or their representative the right to challenge legally the deprivation of liberty
- providing a system that allows the deprivation of liberty to be reviewed and monitored.

## Examples of deprivation of liberty[4]
- A patient being restrained in order to admit them to hospital.
- Medication being given to a person against their will.
- Staff being in complete control over a patient's care or movements for a long period.
- Staff making all decisions about a patient, including choices about assessments, treatment, and visitors.
- Staff deciding whether a patient can be released into the care of others or to live elsewhere.
- Staff refusing to discharge a patient into the care of others.
- Staff restricting a patient's access to their friends or family.

### The deprivation of liberty authorization process[5]

Once a supervisory body receives a deprivation of liberty application they must arrange an assessment within 21 days that seeks to ensure the conditions for a deprivation of liberty are met. These include:

- Age—check that the person is over 18 years old.
- Mental health—decide whether the person has a mental disorder.
- Mental capacity—check that the person lacks capacity.
- Best interests—check that the deprivation of liberty is in the person's best interest to safeguard them from harm, or the reasonable likelihood of harm.
- Eligibility—assess whether the person meets the requirement for detention under the Mental Health Act. If they do, a deprivation of liberty authorization is not appropriate
- No refusals—check whether any advance decisions are in place, and also whether the authorization conflicts with decisions made by a court order.

### References

3  National Institute for Health and Care Excellence (NICE). *Self-Harm: the short-term physical and psychological management and secondary prevention of self-harm in primary and secondary care.* CG16. NICE: London, 2004. ℘ www.nice.org.uk/guidance/cg16/informationforpublic
4  Alzheimer's Society. *Deprivation of Liberty Safeguards (DoLS).* ℘ www.alzheimers.org.uk/site/scripts/documents_info.php?documentID=1327
5  *Mental Capacity Act 2005.* ℘ www.legislation.gov.uk/ukpga/2005/9/contents

# Index

# Mental Health (Care and Treatment) (Scotland) Act 2003

| Section/Part | Duration | Mental Welfare Commission (MWC)/ Mental Health Tribunal (MHT) | Appeal | Consent |
|---|---|---|---|---|
| 36<br>Emergency detention in hospital | 72 hours | MWC informed if Mental Health Officer (MHO) consent not obtained | No<br>Can be revoked by Approved Medical Practitioner | MHO, where practicable |
| 44<br>Short-term detention in hospital | 28 days<br>Can be extended by 3 days prior to CTO | MWC/MHT to be informed within 7 days | Patient/ named person can apply to Tribunal for revocation of certificate | MHO<br>Named person to be informed |
| 299<br>Nurse's holding power | 2 hours<br>Can be extended by 1 hour to allow examination to be carried out | MWC to be informed in writing | No | No |
| Part 7<br>Compulsory Treatment Order (CTO)<br>Treatment enforced either in hospital or community setting | 6 months, followed by 6 months, then 12 monthly | Tribunal makes decision on application | At time of Tribunal hearing and after 3 months | No |
| Interim CTO<br>When further assessment required prior to applying CTO | 28 days, further 28 days, maximum 56 days | Tribunal makes decision | At time of Tribunal hearing | No |
| 112<br>Detention in event of failure to attend for treatment under CTO | 6 hours | MHO consulted | No | MHO consent required |
| 130<br>Assessment of mentally disordered offenders | 28 days | Responsible Medical Officer (RMO) must report to court before end of 28 days | No | No |
| 133<br>Compulsion Order<br>For mentally disordered offenders | 6 months but under regular review by RMO | RMO must report to court if order no longer appropriate | No | No |
| 134<br>Detention of acquitted persons for assessment | 6 hours | MWC to be informed within 7 days | No | No |

## The Mental Health Act 2007 (England)

| Section number and purpose | Maximum duration | Can patient apply to Mental Health Review Tribunal (MHRT)? | Automatic MHRT hearing? | Can nearest relative apply to MHRT? | Do consent to treatment issues apply? |
|---|---|---|---|---|---|
| 2<br>Admission for assessment – application may be made by the nearest relative or an Approved Mental Health Professional (AMHP), and supported by two medical recommendations | 28 days, not renewable | Within first 14 days | No | No | Yes |
| 3<br>Admission for treatment – application may be made by a nearest relative or an AMHP, supported by two medical recommendations | 6 months<br>May be renewed for 6 months, then annually | Within first 6 months, then in each period | Yes – at 6 months, then every 3 years (yearly if under 16) if no application | No | Yes |
| 4<br>Emergency admission for assessment made by at least one medical recommendation | 72 hours<br>Not renewable but 2nd medical recommendation can change to s2 | Yes, but only if s4 is converted to s2 | No | No | No |
| 5(2)<br>Doctor's or Approved Clinician's holding power | 72 hours<br>Not renewable | No | No | No | No |
| 5(4)<br>Nurse's holding power | 6 hours<br>Not renewable, but doctor or Approved Clinician can change to s5(2) | No | No | No | No |